The Chronic Fatigue Cure: The Most Comprehensive Book on The Many Causes and Treatments for Chronic Fatigue

Dr. Susan's Healthy Living
drsusasnshealthyliving.com

Facebook.com/DrSusanRichards
drsusanshealthyliving@gmail.com
(650) 561-9978

ISBN 978-1511961769

Note

The information in this book is meant to complement the advice and guidance of your physician, not replace it. It is very important that any person who has medical problems be evaluated by a physician. If you are under the care of a physician, you should discuss any major changes in your regimen with him or her. Because this is a book and not a medical consultation, keep in mind that the information presented here may not apply in your particular case. In view of individual medical requirements, new research, and government regulations, it is the responsibility of the reader to validate health practices and treatments with a physician or health service.

Table of Contents

Introduction

Dear Friend,

I am thrilled that you have found my book, *The Chronic Fatigue Cure*, because I know that you are looking for positive and effective solutions to heal from this issue. I have written this book just for you, to share with you the all-natural treatment program that I have developed for my own patients who were also suffering from the debilitating effects caused by chronic fatigue and tiredness.

Over the years I have worked with many women patients who have complained of fatigue. In fact, fatigue is one of the most common reasons why women visit their physicians. My patients with chronic fatigue have told me that they were finding it difficult to get through the day and do their errands and responsibilities, handle the demands of their careers, jobs and families. Some of my patients with severe chronic fatigue actually had to quit their jobs and go on disability because they couldn't make it through the day.

Fatigue is a common complaint for many health problems including chronic fatigue syndrome/myalgic encephalomyelitis, fibromyalgia, depression, prolonged stress, weak adrenal glands, anemia, low thyroid condition, allergies, menopause, and PMS. larkIf these tests are negative, they may throw up their hands and imply that it's all due to stress or "it's all in your head" and the patient remains undiagnosed and untreated.

A Self-Help Guide to Chronic Fatigue

Though fatigue in itself will not kill a person, it can tremendously lower the quality of life and functional ability of people affected by it. My patients have come to me looking for solutions that would really work and would help restore their energy, vitality and elevate their mood. When experiencing prolonged fatigue and tiredness, it is difficult to organize and carry through with your activities. This can hamper effective performance in many different areas of life. You may also be struggling with these issues, too and are searching for solutions.

I want to share with you the stories of three women who came to me as patients. They each had a different health issue, yet were all struggling with fatigue and exhaustion. I was able to successfully treat all of these women using my treatment programs, enabling them to regain their energy and vitality and restore a positive and optimistic mood. These stories illustrate how prevalent fatigue is as a major symptom in many different conditions.

Linda's Story

When I saw Linda as a patient, she told me that she had "run out of steam." She was so tired and exhausted from years of stress, both in her marriage which had finally ended in divorce and stress on the job, that she was too tired to even work. She had already cut her work schedule and was now concerned that she would have to go on disability. Her laboratory tests hadn't found any particular illness; she was just very depleted so there was nothing much that her physicians could do for her. Her physician had recommended antidepressant medication, which she tried for a few weeks. But it had significant and very unpleasant side effects and she discontinued taking the two drugs immediately. She was profoundly depressed by her situation and felt that she had no hope.

She needed to have an evaluation done that pinpointed her weak adrenal function and brain chemistry imbalances. Her poor dietary and nutritional habits were also contributing to fatigue and burnout. I started her on a powerful and effective anti-fatigue program including vitamins, minerals, amino acids and herbs that significantly helped to boost her energy along with my anti-fatigue diet. She also began a stress reduction program to repattern her emotional stress responses and restore peace, joy and positivity in her life. She found that day by day, her energy was returning and that she was able to return more and more to her normal schedule. This was a profound relief to her. She considered her renewed level of energy a healing miracle!

Carole's Story

Carole came to see me as a patient because she had been struggling with depression and tiredness for many years. She shared with me that this issue was a family pattern and that close relatives, including her father, had also struggled with severe depression. She had periods where she became reclusive and wouldn't even socialize with friends and her family due to her mood issues.

She would sometimes spend days locked up in her house, sitting on her couch feeling very exhausted, bleak and depressed about her life even though she had caring friends, and two grown children who loved her. She refused to consider antidepressant medication and, unfortunately, did not get enough relief from a nutritional supplement program that she tried to put together on her own to really shift her mood.

I started Carole on a program that included my anti-fatigue diet and a very effective nutritional supplement program to help bring her brain chemistry into better balance and help shift her mood and restore her energy. She was also an excellent candidate for red light therapy, which is a very exciting treatment for fatigue, lack of energy, mood imbalances and fibromyalgia.

Carole also began to take daily walks, which is very beneficial for relieving depression. She also began to do an emotional repatterning program that I suggested to her. Thankfully, her mood began to lighten and her depression started to lift. Within a few weeks she told me that she was feeling quite a bit better.

Alice's Story

Alice came to see me as a patient because of her pain and chronic fatigue symptoms due to fibromyalgia. Here is how Alice, described her symptoms due to this condition,

"I've really been suffering terribly from the ill effects of this condition. I have a great deal of aches and pains in my muscles, and I suffer from frequent muscle spasms. I feel stiff most of the time, which is really challenging for me since my job requires me to sit at a computer for eight hours a day. I also have trouble sleeping, and I wake up repeatedly during the night and I feel exhausted all day. Worst of all are my frequent and unbearable headaches. My doctor has prescribed anti-inflammatory medication, but this hasn't been very effective. I'm hoping that you can help me find more effective natural treatments to relieve my symptoms."

Alice was thrilled as her chronic pain, muscle spasms, stiffness and fatigue began to resolve as she followed my program. She was very eager and motivated to gain relief from her symptoms. A combination of dietary changes, a targeted nutritional supplement program, meditation and breathing exercises along with an exercise program of gentle stretches and walking as well as red light therapy proved to be very beneficial in restoring her energy and relieving her pain and discomfort.

Happily, I have seen dramatic and positive results for many of my patients, like the three that I have shared with you, with my anti-fatigue programs. It has been very exciting for me to see thousands of women regain their energy, strength, vitality, optimism and joy of living. I have always loved working with my patients as a team effort and it has reaped great results! My patients have been thrilled with the terrific benefits that they received from following my program and I am delighted to be sharing this program with you. This book is filled with much practical and useful information and I look forward to you receiving great benefits, too.

Although women with chronic fatigue and tiredness should have their underlying medical problems diagnosed and treated, you cannot underestimate the importance of practicing beneficial lifestyle habits to regain a high level of energy, whether you use medical treatments or not. All women with chronic fatigue can benefit from lifestyle based self-care treatment programs.

I have researched the use of therapeutic anti-fatigue diets, nutritional supplement programs, light therapy and many other techniques that support optimal health and help treat the various causes of chronic fatigue. I have worked with specific stretches and exercise programs, acupressure points as well as emotional repatterning programs and stress management techniques to provide my patients with a variety of effective self-care treatment options. I have also worked with medications, where necessary and appropriate, to give my patients the treatments that would most assist in their recovery

How to Use This Book

I feel strongly that any woman interested in healing from fatigue and tiredness and regaining her energy, vitality and joy of living should have access to this information. Because there are many women whom I will never see as patients in my medical practice, I wrote this book to share the program that I have developed and found, through years of medical practice, to be most useful. I hope you will find this information as useful as my patients have. I am continuously expanding my own knowledge about the most up-to-date therapies and researching new healthcare techniques for treating this issue.

My program includes my two part anti-fatigue diet, delicious menus, meal plans and recipes as well as the vitamins, minerals, essential fatty acids, amino acids and herbs that I have found to be the most effective in eliminating my patient's symptoms and restoring their energy and vitality.

I also share with you wonderful techniques to help increase your energy through positive repatterning of your emotions and feelings as well as meditations, affirmations, visualizations and deep breathing exercises that promote energy, joy and relaxation. I have included acupressure massage points, stretching exercises and recommendations for physical exercise that are specifically helpful for the relief of fatigue and tiredness.

The book contains important chapters on the symptoms, risk factors and diagnosis of the major medical issues linked to chronic fatigue. I also discuss the most up-to-date drug therapies for these medical conditions and explain the pros and cons of all the medical treatments.

I recommend that you read through the entire book first to familiarize yourself with the material. The Chronic Fatigue Workbook will help you evaluate your symptoms, risk factors, and fatigue-creating lifestyle habits.

Next, turn to the therapy chapters and read through the self-care treatments of the book. Try the therapies that most appeal to you and pertain to your symptoms. Establish a regimen that works for you and follow it every day.

My chronic fatigue healing program is practical and easy to follow. You may use it by itself or in conjunction with a medical program. While working with a physician may be necessary to establish a definitive diagnosis of the causes of fatigue, and medical therapy may be important for treatable conditions like thyroid disease, my self-care program will provide you with very beneficial support to restore your energy and vitality and then maintain them. The material contained in this book will not only help speed up the diagnostic process but will bring you significant relief.

My treatment program can play a major role in reducing your fatigue symptoms and preventing their recurrence. The feelings of radiant energy and wellness that can be yours with this self-care program will radiate out and touch your whole life. I hope that your life is positively transformed by these beneficial therapies.

Love,

Dr. Susan

Part I:
Identifying the Problem

1

What Is Chronic Fatigue?

I want to begin our journey together of supporting your healing from chronic fatigue and tiredness by giving you important information about how fatigue can affect a woman's life and the conditions that have most frequently been linked to this symptom. These conditions cover the gamut from physical, psychological and emotional causes of fatigue. This will help you to better understand your fatigue-related symptoms and what might be triggering them. I also discuss the chemical and physiological imbalances that can occur with fatigue and tiredness.

Chronic fatigue is one of the most common complaints physicians hear. In at least twenty percent of all medical visits, patients name fatigue as a significant symptom. Millions of people function below par, accepting chronic fatigue and tiredness as a way of life. They never seek medical care because they think fatigue is a burden that they simply must endure.

In my practice, many of the women seeking help are so tired that they have difficulty carrying out their day-to-day functions. My patients often tell me that their lack of energy seriously affects their quality of life. Many women find it hard to get up and get going from the moment the alarm rings in the morning.

For these women, doing their daily tasks at work or even interacting with friends and family may be difficult. Many of my patients also complain of losing steam and tiring in the afternoon. Once this fatigue sets in, it may pursue a woman until she drops into an exhausted sleep at bedtime. When seeing a new patient, fatigue is one of the first complaints that I address, because sufficient energy is central to day-to-day functioning.

Fatigue has many causes. It is a component of many of the most common health problems affecting women. In this book, I have chosen to focus on the health conditions affecting the four body systems that are most likely to be the cause of fatigue and tiredness. These can include:

- The **immune system** fights foreign invaders in the body, such as bacteria, viruses, and cancer cells
- The **brain** and **nervous system** is comprised of the brain which controls all of our thoughts, feelings and mental and physical functions as well as the fibers that connect the brain, organs, and muscles by transmitting impulses that allow normal bodily sensation and movement. The experience and expression of moods and feelings are also regulated by chemicals produced within the brain.
- The **endocrine or glandular system** regulates reproductive and metabolic functions, such as menstruation and the efficient burning of food for energy. The endocrine glands communicate with one another by secreting into the bloodstream chemicals called hormones that carry chemical messages from one gland to another.
- The **hematological system** is responsible for forming red blood cells, which carry oxygen to all tissues of the body, and white blood cells, which fight infections and other invaders in the body.

The remainder of this chapter discusses problems that arise in these systems—problems in which fatigue is a significant symptom.

The Immune System

Chronic Fatigue Syndrome/Myalgic Encephalomyelitis (ME/CFS)

One of the most publicized causes of fatigue today, chronic fatigue syndrome (CFS) affects over 1 million Americans. It is thought that millions more are affected by this severe and disabling problem but are undiagnosed.

Chronic fatigue syndrome is also referred to as myalgic encephalomyelitis. Let me define what this long term means. Myalgic refers to muscle pain or tenderness while encephalomyelitis means an inflammatory condition of the brain and spinal cord. ME/CFS is now recognized as part of a range of illnesses in which fatigue and tiredness are major symptoms.

Women predominate among persons affected with ME/CFS, in fact, 75 percent of the cases are female. Symptoms must last at least 6 months in order to have the diagnosis of this condition. Fatigue is the most prevalent symptom, occurring in almost all the afflicted. The onset of fatigue is often sudden, and many women can pinpoint when it started. The fatigue is so severe that even minor exertion, such as a short walk or light housework, can be debilitating. The loss of physical stamina and endurance is pronounced in women with ME/CFS. Many women with this issue curtail their activities and take naps during the day or sleep more hours at night. Interestingly, increased bed rest doesn't improve the energy level of afflicted women.

ME/CFS occurs with a whole range of other symptoms, including headaches, tender and enlarged lymph nodes, sore throat, loss of memory and poor ability to concentrate and decreased mental acuity, muscle pain, joint aches and pains that move from one joint to another without swelling or redness and unrefreshing sleep. Other common symptoms include depression, anxiety and panic attacks, dizziness or fainting, irritable bowel, chills and night sweats, allergies, digestive complaints and weight loss.

For many women, mental and emotional symptoms seem to predominate. The rate of depression is very high in women with CFS as well as decreased mental acuity. Short-term memory may be diminished. Women with ME/CFS often have trouble remembering specific names or places, or doing complex mental work, such as bookkeeping, administrative tasks, or teaching. Thus, women with ME/CFS may have great difficulty performing functions that demand intellectual skills.

The cause of ME/CFS is still unknown. No primary cause has been found that is consistent for all cases of this condition. There are no blood tests or other laboratory tests or scans that can definitely diagnose this condition.

Many experts now believe that ME/CFS develops from a combination of different factors that may include:

- Viral or other infections
- Genetic defects
- Overactive immune system
- Multiple chemical sensitivities
- Brain chemistry abnormalities
- Hormone imbalances
- Stress related or emotional conditions.

Because many symptoms of ME/CFS resemble those of a viral infection, much attention from researchers has focused on the possibility that a virus or other pathogen causes these symptoms, at least in some cases. Most of the attention has focused on the herpes family of viruses as the causative agents. These include the Epstein-Barr virus (EBV), herpesvirus type 6 (HHV-6) and human T cell lymphotropic virus (HTLV) but none of these has emerged as a cause of ME/CFS. Environmental pollutants or contaminants may also play a role in weakening the body and allowing ME/CFS to develop.

Other researchers have linked ME/CFS to brain neurotransmitter and hormonal imbalances. Some patients have been found to have high levels of serotonin, the inhibitory neurotransmitter, and low levels of dopamine and dopamine that promote energy and zest for life. These findings would be consistent with chronic fatigue and depression. In addition some patients appear to have low levels of cortisol, the adrenal stress hormone that would normally provide resistance to infections, psychological stress and exercise. In some patients with ME/CFS, they appear to have disturbed circadian rhythm that causes a disturbance of the sleep-wake cycle. None of these imbalances, however, seem to be useful for routine screening and testing for ME/CFS.

Many of my ME/CFS patients report extreme and prolonged emotional stress, anxiety, and depression, and a history of poor nutritional habits predating the onset of ME/CFS. The length of the illness varies. While some ME/CFS patients recover fairly quickly, most continue to remain ill longer than two years. I have seen patients in my practice for which ME/CFS has been a long-term and extremely debilitating condition. These women had tried many drugs and natural treatment regimens. In treating women with ME/CFS, I have had success with my patients in combining a variety of supportive techniques, primarily in the self-care or lifestyle area. I describe these techniques fully in the following chapters.

The Nervous System

Depression

Depression is characterized as feeling so down or "blue" that these feelings interfere with daily life, including one's job and family life. No amount of "cheering up" or trying to tough your way through it can make it go away. If you are clinically depressed you are likely to be suffering from feelings of sadness, emptiness and hopelessness about your current life situation and the future. Almost 15 million American adults are affected by depression each year, including twice as many women as men. It is estimated that 30 million people suffer from depression during their lifetime.

If you are depressed, you are likely to suffer from a variety of symptoms that cause you to feel lethargic, fatigued, and unable to cope with other people and normal life activities. These symptoms include difficulty in concentrating and making decisions, and lack of self-esteem and self-confidence. Depressed women may suffer from a feeling of worthlessness, guilt and self-pity and may want to isolate themselves from other people to avoid social contact.

Women with depression and sadness can also display anxiety and irritability. They often suffer from eating problems (either overeating or under eating), insomnia, fatigue, digestive complaints, loss of sex drive, headaches, and backaches. Most dangerous to the women affected is that severe depression can lead to suicide attempts. Any threat of suicide in a depressed woman should be taken seriously and immediate medical care begun.

Brain chemistry imbalances, especially in the inhibitory and excitatory neurotransmitters, can lead to depression. Let's look more closely at how these neurotransmitters function in the brain to help you understand better how depression can occur.

Serotonin and dopamine are two of our main neurotransmitters. These are naturally occurring chemicals that relay electrical messages between nerve cells throughout your body. Serotonin is part of the inhibitory pathway, while dopamine is part of the excitatory pathway. Because these two pathways oppose and complement one another, imbalances in either serotonin or dopamine can make a person more sensitive to everyday stress than someone who is able to produce these neurochemicals in more balanced and appropriate amounts.

The action of serotonin on the nerves is inhibitory, thus it helps to relieve stress and calms the mind. Serotonin also regulates appetite, influences mood, and promotes deep, peaceful sleep and healthy hormone production.

Dopamine is a neurotransmitter that stimulates and energizes the body. In fact, dopamine is actually a precursor to substances made by the adrenal medulla and sympathetic nervous system that can trigger the stress response within the body when you are under duress. High levels of dopamine have been linked to such traits as mental alertness, physical energy, and vitality, as well as aggressive drive and libido.

Dopamine is synthesized by the adrenal glands and is converted by the body into the stress hormones epinephrine and norepinephrine, which also stimulate hormone production. Before ages 40–45, dopamine levels remain fairly stable, but they then decrease by about 13 percent per decade.

As levels of these neurotransmitters begin to decline with age, your body's ability to handle stressful events can change. Depressed serotonin levels can trigger mood imbalances, sleeplessness, and food cravings. For example, women who suffer from PMS may have a tendency towards low serotonin levels. That's one reason why women with PMS often respond to stressful events in an exaggerated manner.

Irritability, anger, tension, and upset are common responses in the second half of the menstrual cycle to such usually small stresses as a nagging child, a minor disagreement with a spouse, or a work deadline. Women with low serotonin may be tired and exhausted from insomnia and lack of sleep.

In contrast, when levels of the stimulatory neurotransmitter dopamine are depressed, epinephrine and norepinephrine production is also diminished. This is more common in women who are frequently fatigued, tired, lethargic, and lack vital force and joy of life, and depression.

As a result, imbalances in both inhibitory and excitatory neurotransmitters can predispose you to depression and fatigue. Many of my patients with chronic fatigue and depression suffer from neurotransmitter imbalances since these two symptoms often go hand in hand. Correcting these imbalances is the basis on which the most frequently prescribed antidepressant drugs work.

Many stressful life events can also lead to depression, including death of a loved one, divorce, loss of a job, or even aging. Women who are experiencing low thyroid conditions, PMS, menopause, or the postpartum period are at higher risk of depression. Poor nutritional habits or the use of drugs and hormones (such as hormone replacement therapy for menopause and birth control pills) can add to depression. Some women with depression are sensitive to the change of seasons. The shortness of the days and decreased light during the winter can trigger depression because the endocrine system may need more daylight to function optimally.

Women with depression may need a combination of antidepressant medication along with psychotherapy to combat the condition. Self-care techniques such as exercise, therapeutic diet, nutritional supplementation and stress management can also be very helpful.

Fibromyalgia

Fibromyalgia is condition that has also been linked to neurotransmitter imbalances, specifically low inhibitory neurotransmitters like serotonin as well as psychological, genetic, environmental, nutritional and other factors. It is considered to be a syndrome with a number of signs and symptoms that occur together but without an identifiable cause. (In contrast, a disease often has a specific, recognizable cause.)

The list of symptoms linked to fibromyalgia is long and can vary from woman to woman. The most common symptoms of fibromyalgia are at least six months of widespread chronic pain, muscle spasm and tightness, fatigue and sleep disturbances like insomnia and waking up feeling tired. Other symptoms include generalized aches and stiffness upon waking up or staying in one position for too long and numbness and tingling in the face, arms, hands, legs or feet.

Fibromyalgia sufferers also have a heightened and painful response to pressure. They are hypersensitive to touch and experience pain in at least 11 out of 18 characteristic tender points. These are places on your body where slight pressure causes pain.

Some of these tender points on the body can include:

- The front of the throat just above the collarbone
- The back of the head at the base of the skull
- Just below the front of the collarbone
- Upper back between the neck and shoulders
- Upper back between the shoulder blades
- Inner crease of the elbows
- Where the buttocks meet the back
- On the inside of the knee joint

They may also experience chronic tension or migraine headaches, jaw and facial tenderness, sensitivity to odors, bright lights, loud noise, certain foods and medications, difficulty concentrating, memory issues, heart palpitations and vertigo. Irritable bowel and bladder symptoms can occur and include abdominal pain, bloating, nausea, constipation alternating with diarrhea and urinary frequency or urgency. Fibromyalgia often coexists with psychological conditions such as depression, anxiety and posttraumatic stress disorder.

Fibromyalgia is estimated to affect 3 to 5 percent of the population, or six to ten million people, mostly women. In fact, women are more affected than men by a 9 to 1 ratio. It can be a frustrating condition for many women to deal with because its underlying cause is still a mystery. As a result, there's no definitive test for fibromyalgia and the diagnosis is made by a process of elimination.

There are many theories, however, as to what chemical and physical imbalances in the body may be triggering fibromyalgia symptoms. Some researchers have speculated that fibromyalgia may be linked to lower levels of the brain inhibitory neurotransmitter, serotonin. Healthy serotonin levels normally have a calming and relaxing effect on your mood and body. It also helps to reduce anxiety and your reactivity to stress. When serotonin levels are diminished, it leads to lowered pain thresholds as well as an increased sensitivity to pain.

The increased sensitivity to pain seen with fibromyalgia sufferers may also be due to a reduced effectiveness of endorphins, the body's natural painkillers as well as an increase in a chemical called substance P that amplifies pain signals.

Some studies link fibromyalgia to sudden trauma causing stress to the brain and spinal cord. Research published in the Journal of Neural Transmission has found actual physical changes in the structure of the frontal, motor and cingulate cortices of the brain in fibromyalgia patients.

Many women develop fibromyalgia within a year after undergoing a complete hysterectomy or following the onset of menopause. Sometimes symptoms begin after surgery, physical trauma or significant psychological stress that causes post-traumatic stress disorder. Sometimes, infections appear to trigger or worsen fibromyalgia. There may also be a genetic component for some women since fibromyalgia tends to run in families. Thus, there may be genetic mutations that may make you more susceptible to developing this condition.

In summary, while no single factor has emerged as being the definitive cause of fibromyalgia, most researchers believe that fibromyalgia results not from a single event but from a combination of many physical, chemical and emotional triggers.

As often happens with a disorder that the medical community doesn't fully understand, conventional medical treatment involves prescribing a wide-variety of medications that can include anti-inflammatories, muscle relaxants, antidepressants, tranquilizers, anticonvulsants and sleeping pills. While these drugs can help to numb the pain, they don't heal the underlying issues that may be causing the pain in the first place. In the self-care chapters of this book, you will find a number of very beneficial therapies that can help to eliminate the painful fibromyalgia symptoms and bring your body back into a healthier balance.

Endocrine or Glandular System

Premenstrual Syndrome (PMS)

Mood swings, irritability, fatigue and depression are frequently encountered symptoms of premenstrual syndrome (PMS). PMS is one of the most common problems affecting women during their reproductive years (from the teens to the early fifties). In fact, it affects one-third to one-half of American women in this age group. In my practice, more than 90 percent of women with PMS complain of mood swings, irritability, fatigue, depression and sadness that increases in intensity varying from several days to the week or two prior to menstruation.

Many PMS patients describe mood and personality changes that occur during this time. Even if they are normally calm and patient, they may become irritable and more moody as their menstrual period approaches. They often feel more blue and depressed, reacting with tears to things that would never trigger these feelings during their PMS-free time of the month. My patients have told me that they are impatient and irritable with their children, pick fights with their spouses, and snap at friends and co-workers. Some spend the rest of the month repairing the emotional damage done to their relationships during this time.

In addition to the emotional symptoms, PMS has numerous physical symptoms involving almost every system in the body. More than 150 symptoms have been documented, including headaches, bloating, breast tenderness, weight gain, sugar craving, and acne. However, for many women, the emotional symptoms and fatigue are the most severe, adversely affecting their family relationships and their ability to work. In addition, it is not unusual for women to have as many as 10 to 12 of the symptoms.

There is no single hormonal or chemical imbalance that has been linked to PMS. Instead, over two dozen hormonal, nutritional and chemical imbalances may contribute to causing the symptoms. Even more confusing for patients and physicians alike is that the underlying causes may differ from one woman to another. Though it is not entirely known what causes the moodiness, irritability, fatigue and depression symptoms, research suggests that several types of imbalances are likely culprits.

One possible cause is an imbalance in the body's estrogen and progesterone levels. Both estrogen and progesterone increase during the second half of the menstrual cycle. Their chemical actions affect the function of almost every organ system in the body. When properly balanced, estrogen and progesterone promote healthy and balanced emotions.

However, PMS mood symptoms may occur if the balance between these hormones is abnormal, because they have an opposing effect on the chemistry of the brain. Estrogen acts as a natural mood elevator and stimulant while progesterone has a sedative effect on the nervous system. If estrogen predominates, women tend to feel anxious; and if progesterone predominates, women tend to feel depressed and tired.

Other examples of the opposing effects of estrogen and progesterone include the following: estrogen lowers blood sugar, progesterone elevates it; estrogen promotes synthesis of fats in the tissues, progesterone breaks them down. Thus, when estrogen and progesterone are appropriately balanced, women are more likely to have normal mood and behavioral patterns.

The balance between these hormones depends on two things: how much hormone the body produces, and how efficiently the body breaks it down and disposes of it. The ovaries are the primary source of estrogen and progesterone in premenopausal women (with estrogen also being synthesized by intestinal bacteria and by conversion of adrenal hormones to estrogen by the fatty tissues). The liver has the major responsibility for breaking down and inactivating estrogen. The liver tries to make sure the levels of estrogen circulating through the body in a chemically active form don't become too high.

Breakdown in the liver's ability to perform this function affects the levels of estrogen, as well as other hormones, in the body. Both emotional stress and your nutritional habits play significant roles in how efficiently this system will run. For example, excessive intake of fats, alcohol, and sugar stresses the liver, which must process these foods as well as the hormone.

With vitamin B deficiency, which can be caused by poor nutrition or by emotional stress, the liver lacks the raw material to carry out its metabolic tasks. In either case, the liver cannot break down the hormones efficiently, so higher levels of hormones continue to circulate in the blood without proper disposal. This can worsen the moodiness, fatigue and depression seen with PMS.

Other research studies link the emotional symptoms of PMS to chemical imbalances in the brain and central nervous system. Some researchers suggest that the symptoms of anxiety and mood swings are due to a heightened sensitivity in some women to fluctuations in the body's level of beta-endorphins. These substances are the body's natural opiates, producing a sense of well-being and even elation when present in large amounts. (Beta-endorphins are responsible for the "runner's high" that many people experience after prolonged aerobic exercise, because exercise increases beta-endorphin production.)

Beta-endorphin levels increase soon after ovulation at mid-cycle and may decline with the approach of menstruation. A fall in beta-endorphin levels in women who are very sensitive to the effects of these chemicals or who produce large amounts of beta-endorphins could, like opiate withdrawal, cause symptoms such as fatigue and tiredness.

Another possible cause of PMS anxiety symptoms may be the lack of sufficient serotonin in the brain. As discussed earlier in this chapter, serotonin is a neurotransmitter that regulates rapid eye movement (REM) sleep and appetite. Inadequate levels of serotonin could explain the poor sleep quality with the resultant fatigue, moodiness and irritability from which some women with PMS suffer.

It could also explain, at least in part, why some women with PMS feel that they have such a difficult time controlling their eating habits and managing their food cravings during the premenstrual time. Serotonin is produced in the body from an amino acid called tryptophan. Tryptophan is an essential amino acid that must be replaced daily through adequate dietary intake since our body cannot manufacture it from other sources. Good sources of tryptophan include almonds, pumpkin seeds, and sesame seeds.

Many factors increase the risk of PMS in susceptible women. PMS occurs most frequently in women over 30, in fact, the most severe symptoms often occur in women in their thirties and forties. Women are at high risk when they are under significant emotional stress or if they have poor nutritional habits and don't exercise. Women who are unable to tolerate birth control pills seem to be more likely to suffer PMS, as are women who have had a pregnancy complicated by toxemia. Also, the more children a woman has, the more severe her PMS symptoms.

PMS rarely goes away spontaneously without treatment. My experience is that it gets worse with age. Some of my most uncomfortable patients are women in their middle to late forties who are approaching menopause. These women often feel they have the worst of both life phases as they pass from their reproductive years into menopause. Often, PMS symptoms coexist with bleeding irregularities and hot flashes in premenopausal women that can both worsen fatigue. Once the PMS is treated, the accompanying fatigue and mood symptoms clear up. Therapies for PMS are discussed in the self-help section of this book.

Since no individual hormonal or chemical imbalance has been linked to PMS, there is no single wonder drug that cures PMS, although many drugs have been tested. These include hormones, tranquilizers, antidepressants, and diuretics with varying degrees of success. Luckily, the mood swings, irritability, fatigue and depression symptoms of PMS as well as the physical symptoms respond very well to healthful lifestyle changes.

In my clinical practice, I have found PMS to be a very treatable problem. I have had great success with my PMS relief program. A therapeutic diet, the use of nutritional supplements, a stress management program and other self-care therapies are very effective in eliminating PMS symptoms.

Menopause

Menopause, the end of menstrual bleeding, occurs for most women between the ages of 48 and 52. However, some women cease menstruating as young as their late thirties or early forties, while others continue to menstruate into their mid-fifties. Fatigue and tiredness often accompanies this process as women go through the decrease in female hormone production that lead to the cessation of menstruation.

For most women, the transition to menopause occurs gradually, triggered by a slowdown in the function of their ovaries. The process begins four to six years before the last menstrual period and continues for several years after. During this period of transition, estrogen production from the ovaries decreases, finally dropping to such low levels that menstruation becomes irregular and finally ceases entirely. For some women this transition to a new, lower level of hormonal equilibrium is easy and uneventful.

For many women, however, the transition is difficult and fraught with many uncomfortable symptoms, such as irregular bleeding, hot flashes, mood swings, depression and fatigue. As many as 80 percent of all women going through menopause experience hot flashes and other symptoms like insomnia, sleep disturbances, fatigue, depression, low sex drive and vaginal dryness are very common..

One of the most uncomfortable symptoms of menopause are hot flashes—sudden and intense sensations of heat that occur unexpectedly. A woman suddenly notices that she feels warm, and often experiences heavy sweating. As the sweating cools her skin temperature, she begins to shiver. In response to this uncomfortable fluctuation in temperature, many women alternately shed and add clothes. Hot flashes frequently begin on the chest, neck, or face, and radiate to other parts of the body.

While eighty percent of women in menopause experience hot flashes, 40 percent of these women have symptoms severe enough to seek medical care. Hot flashes may occur during both day and night. When they occur at night, they can interrupt a woman's sleep pattern, leaving her exhausted and fatigued during the day from sleep deprivation. Though most flashes appear to occur without any specific environmental trigger, coffee and alcohol intake may spark a flash. The frequency, intensity, and duration of hot flashes vary greatly. For most women they last two or three minutes, but they can last longer, even up to an hour in some cases. In most women, the symptoms begin to subside within four to six years after the last menstrual period.

Vaginal infections may become more frequent because the tissues are easily traumatized. The changes that occur in the urethral tissues may increase the frequency of urination. Women find that they have to get up at night to void, which—like hot flashes—can interrupt sleep and worsen fatigue. Even more frustrating for some women is the tendency to leak urine when they laugh, sneeze, or cough.

Besides the physical changes, many women may note mild to marked changes in their moods during menopause. These symptoms include depression, anxiety, mood swings and irritability. Both estrogen and progesterone have been studied for their effects on mood. Estrogen has a mood elevating effect while progesterone has a calming effect on mood. If estrogen predominates, women tend to feel anxious; if progesterone predominates, women may feel depressed and tired.

With a decrease in both hormones, symptoms can run the gamut from irritability to fatigue and depression. The severity of the symptoms probably depends on the woman's individual biochemistry, as well as social factors. Women have worse symptoms if they are under severe emotional stress or have aggravating dietary habits, such as excessive caffeine, sugar, or alcohol intake.

Many effective treatments, such as bioidentical hormone replacement therapy, therapeutic diet and the use of vitamin, herbal, and mineral supplements, help support menopausal women's reproductive and endocrine systems. Stress management techniques and regular exercise may also help to restore energy and vitality and stabilize mood. These are discussed in the self-care section of this book.

Weak Adrenals

The adrenal glands are part of our stress response system. The adrenals are two triangular-shaped organs, about the size of almonds, resting on top of each kidney. The adrenal glands secrete several dozen hormones to help us regulate stresses of all types. Stress can be a response to strong emotional feelings, such as anxiety or depression, or to physical triggers, such as prolonged physical exertion, an allergic reaction, infectious disease, burns, surgery, or an accident. You are likely to have weak adrenals......

Each adrenal gland consists of two parts, the medulla, or central section, and the cortex, or outer section. Part of our nervous system called the sympathetic nervous system (SNS) sends nerve impulses into the adrenal medulla causing it to secrete the same type of chemicals as the sympathetic nerves themselves: the hormones epinephrine (commonly referred to as adrenaline) and norepinephrine (or noradrenaline). However, while the SNS secretes these chemicals directly into the tissues, the adrenal medulla secretes them into the bloodstream, which transports them to various target tissues, also in response to stressful situations. Thus, the body has two overlapping systems to manage stress: the production of epinephrine and norepinephrine by both the SNS and the adrenal medulla.

The adrenal cortex, or outer portion of the adrenal gland, also produces hormones that help us to manage physical and chemical stress, called glucocorticoids and mineralocorticoids. Adrenal hormones are primarily produced from acetyl Coenzyme A (acetyl CoA) and cholesterol. Acetyl CoA is a chemical produced in the liver, made from fatty acids and amino acids. Cholesterol is a waxy, white, fatty material, widely distributed in all body cells. The cholesterol in the body is supplied by animal foods in the diet, such as eggs and organ meats, and the liver also produces a certain amount of cholesterol.

Glucocorticoids are especially important in allowing an individual to withstand various kinds of stress. The secretion of cortisol accounts for at least 95 percent of adrenal-glucocorticoid activity. Cortisol is the primary stress hormone. Whatever the source of stress, cortisol lessens its injurious effects on the body, reducing pain, swelling, and fever.

In an attempt to buffer the effects of stress, cortisol is released when the body is threatened by extreme conditions such as infection, intense heat or cold, surgery, and any kind of trauma. Cortisol acts as a natural anti-inflammatory when the body is assaulted by infection, a sports injury, arthritis, or allergy. Cortisol also affects carbohydrate and fat metabolism, promoting the conversion of stored sugars and fat into energy. With extreme and prolonged stress, cortisol levels can remain elevated and create a further source of stress on the body resulting in lack of energy and fatigue.

The mineralocorticoid aldosterone, also produced in the adrenal cortex, has an important role in protecting a person from stress by regulating fluid and electrolyte balance in the body. There must be a correct ratio of sodium and potassium ions inside and outside the cells to maintain normal blood pressure and fluid volume.

When stress has been recurrent and of long duration, the adrenal glands can become exhausted, mustering less and less ability to buffer the negative effects of physical and emotional stress. As a result of adrenal exhaustion, the individual may experience an increase in fatigue and tiredness. If you have weak adrenals, you are likely to be chronically tired and lack the reserve energy needed for intense physical or mental challenges such as taking a rigorous hike or passing a difficult exam, if you are a student.

Women with weak adrenals are more likely to have blood sugar imbalances, like hypoglycemia and allergies, including food allergies. They are also prone to hormonal and menstrual issues like PMS, perimenopausal and menopausal symptoms.

Following a therapeutic diet, taking beneficial nutritional supplements, managing stress and much rest are necessary to restore the adrenals and rebuild the physiological "cushion" to deal with stress. Many helpful treatments listed in the self-care section of this book help to restore the adrenal glands.

Hypothyroidism

Hypothyroidism—an underactive thyroid—is far more common in females than in males. In fact, 90 percent of diagnosed cases are women. Low thyroid condition is a common cause of chronic fatigue and depression and tends to worsen with age. The thyroid affects our energy level because it controls our metabolism (the rate at which our cells burn fuel and oxygen). Women with a slow metabolism caused by an underactive thyroid can suffer from a variety of symptoms.

Besides fatigue, hypothyroid women often complain of a hoarse voice, constipation, intolerance to cold, thickening and scaling of skin, facial puffiness, delay of deep tendon reflexes, and slowness of speech, thought, and movement. They also tend to gain weight easily and find it hard to lose weight on a conventional diet. They may suffer from low blood pressure as well as low blood sugar and may crave carbohydrates.

Clinical diagnosis of hypothyroidism in older women may be difficult because many women do not have the typical symptoms mentioned above. In many older women, debilitation and apathy may be the only signs of low thyroid function. Medical studies suggest that thyroid screening by simple blood tests of thyroid hormones should be a routine part of the physical examination for older patients.

Hypothyroidism is generally treated by thyroid replacement therapy. Older patients may require a much lower maintenance dose of thyroxine than younger women. Self-help aspects of treatment and prevention include taking iodine either in the diet or in supplementary form. According to some evidence, adequate intake of vitamin A, vitamin E, and iodine may be necessary to maintain thyroid health and integrity. Once the underlying thyroid deficiency is treated, many fatigued women notice a rapid improvement in their energy level and vitality.

Women with low thyroid function often have exhaustion in other endocrine glands. The adrenal glands are particularly affected by poor thyroid function, as well as any other physical and emotional stress. The adrenals are two almond-sized glands that secrete several dozen hormones.

Cortisol is an important hormone produced by the adrenal glands that helps regulate our response to stress. Stress can be a response to strong emotional feelings, such as anxiety or depression, or to physical triggers, such as an allergic reaction, infectious disease, burns, surgery, or an accident. Whatever the source of stress, cortisol lessens its injurious effects on the body, reducing pain, swelling, and fever.

When stress has been recurrent and of long duration, the adrenal glands can become exhausted, mustering less and less ability to buffer the negative effects of physical and emotional stress. As a result of adrenal exhaustion, the individual may experience an increase in fatigue and tiredness. Much rest, stress management, and nutritional support is required to restore the adrenals and rebuild the physiological "cushion" to deal with stress. Many helpful techniques listed in the self-help section of this book help to restore the endocrine system.

Additional Immune System

Candida Infections

Although commonly referred to as a yeast, Candida albicans is actually a parasitic fungus. Found most commonly in the large intestine and esophagus, candida is a normal inhabitant of the digestive tract and usually lives in balance with friendly bacteria that help the digestive system function optimally. When the balance between the bacteria and the fungi is upset, candida may proliferate, infecting tissues of the digestive tract, vagina, and mouth. The toxins released by the fungi weaken the immune system, allowing candida to penetrate throughout the body and spread to other systems, such as the bladder and respiratory system.

Women with candida infections in the vagina (candida vaginitis) often have a thick vaginal discharge, redness, itching, and burning. Women with digestive symptoms of candida may have heartburn, bloating, gas, abdominal pain, constipation, and diarrhea. Candida infection of the mouth is called thrush and most commonly afflicts infants and children. Thrush presents with white lesions inside the mouth and on the tongue. In the most severe cases, candida can travel through the bloodstream to invade every organ system in the body. This type of blood poisoning is called candida septicemia and is usually seen only in seriously ill patients, such as people with AIDS or terminal cancer.

The weakening of the immune system caused by the overgrowth of candida has been linked to many symptoms other than those of active infection. These include chronic fatigue, poor ability to concentrate, lethargy, depression, visual changes, pain and swelling in joints, nasal congestion, sore throats, and muscle weakness. Candida infections are more common in diabetics and have been linked to the prolonged use of antibiotics, cortisone, or birth control pills. Diets that include large amounts of bread, alcoholic drinks, candy, cookies, fruit juice, and other foods with high sugar or yeast content promote the growth of candida.

Because candida is present in most people, a candida infection is difficult to diagnose. Women with candida vaginitis may be diagnosed by identifying the organisms on a slide or through taking a medical history of symptoms. Candida can also be diagnosed through a blood test of antibodies to candida or stool analysis However, for women who may have candida in other organ systems and tissues, the most definitive diagnostic test may be their response to a sugar- and yeast-free diet, as well as their response to the appropriate medication. See the treatment section of this book for more information on effective medical and self-care treatment for candida.

Allergies

Many women are unaware that allergic reactions can cause fatigue and depression. In fact, these are common symptoms of an allergic reaction. They can accompany an allergy to foods or to chemical or environmental triggers. Allergy is a very common health issues that affects 20 percent of the population. The number of people with chronic allergy-like symptoms- nasal and chest congestion and cough – but who have nonallergic rhinitis is even higher, affecting one out of three people. It is estimated that the annual cost of allergies to the health care system and businesses is as high as $7.9 billion. Allergies rank 5th among the leading causes of chronic diseases in the U.S. Ten percent of the U.S population suffer from allergies.

Allergies occur when the body's immune system overreacts to harmless substances. Normally, the immune system is on the alert for invaders such as viruses, bacteria, and other organisms that cause disease. The immune system's job is to identify these invaders and to produce antibodies that destroy them before they cause illness. In allergic people, this system begins to react to other substances — typically pollens, molds, or foods such as milk or wheat (called allergens). Common food allergens include wheat, milk (and milk products), alcohol, chocolate, sugar, eggs, yeast, peanuts, citrus fruits, tomatoes, corn, and shellfish.

Food allergies initiate a series of chemical reactions in the body that include the increase in histamine levels that cause inflammations in tissues where allergic symptoms often appear such as the sinuses, lungs and digestive tract. Sometimes allergic reactions are easily diagnosed, because the symptoms occur immediately after the encounter with the allergen.

Immediate allergic symptoms include wheezing, itching and tearing of the eyes, nasal congestion, and hives.

Some allergic reactions are delayed. They may occur hours or days after exposure to the allergen. Delayed symptoms include fatigue, depression, headaches, spaciness, joint aches and pains and eczema. The person affected may be unaware that an allergy is causing her symptoms.

Food allergies can also affect digestive function, causing inflammation of the intestinal lining and pain in the abdominal area. Damage to the intestinal lining causes it to become more porous and permeable. When large particles of poorly digested food, to which the person is allergic, are absorbed into the body, the body's defense system is activated, precipitating damage to many organs and tissues by autoantibodies. (These are the immune complexes that attack your own tissues as if they were foreign substances.) The person affected may be unaware that an allergy is causing her emotional and physical symptoms. This often occurs with food allergies, as well as with a variety of chemical triggers.

Food allergies commonly trigger anxiety episodes in susceptible women. Often, you crave the foods to which you are allergic. Thus, food addiction may actually be a sign of food allergy. Women commonly crave foods such as chocolate, chips, pasta, bread, and milk products. Often they find that once they start eating these foods, they have a difficult time stopping. A woman who has the desire to have one chocolate cookie can end up eating a whole box. The decision to eat one cookie can turn into a binge of ten or fifteen at one session, or a small dish of ice cream becomes a pint.

Though bingeing tendencies can be seen throughout the month in women with food allergies, they tend to be worse during the premenstrual period (which may commence as early as two weeks prior to the onset of menstruation). Alterations in mood, such as depression and fatigue and tiredness can coexist with the food craving symptoms.

Conventional physicians test for food allergies by doing skin tests and blood testing. Unfortunately, these tests are often inaccurate in determining actual food sensitivities. Many people test positively to many healthy foods that they are not allergic to. Some holistic physicians test for food allergies by doing sublingual provocative tests. In this test, a food extract is placed under the tongue to see whether it elicits a reaction. Neutralizing antidotes are then administered to the patient to reduce or eliminate symptoms. This test, however, is not used by traditional allergists.

Finally, there is a blood test called the ELISA (enzyme-linked immuno-absorbent assey) that measures the amount of allergen-specific antibodies in your blood. The advantage of allergy blood testing is that it requires only one needle stick, unlike skin testing. However, this test is more expensive and may not be covered by your health insurance.

One of the easiest ways to test for food sensitivities is simply to eliminate suspected food allergens and over the next month or two see what the affect is on your symptoms. Your doctor may ask you to reintroduce these foods one at a time to see how you react. Many women will find that they feel quite a bit better when they eliminate common allergens like gluten-containing grains such as wheat, dairy products, sugar and soy or other foods to which you suspect you may be allergic. Maintaining a low-stress diet can take a load off of the immune system, allowing both your mood and energy to normalize. During the period when you are determining your food allergies, you may want to keep a diary in which you record your emotional and physical symptoms, both on and off the offending foods, if you try to reintroduce any of them. This will help you evaluate the severity of your reactions.

The conventional treatment for allergies usually includes avoiding the offending substance or using over-the-counter and prescription medication and desensitization shots. Alternative health care doctors are also likely to recommend managing stress and following an elimination diet and nutritional supplement program to help treat and prevent allergies. It is important to rotate foods and choose from a wide variety of high-nutrient food. Certain nutritional supplements help to support and strengthen the immune system. These topics are discussed in the self-care section of this book.

Hematological (Blood-Forming) System

Anemia

Anemia is one of the most common health problems affecting women of all ages and is often a cause of fatigue and tiredness. 12 percent percent of women of child-bearing age have anemia and 20 percent of pregnant women. 10 percent of people over 65 years of age are anemic. Women who are anemic have a reduced number of red cells circulating in their blood or a reduced amount of hemoglobin (the oxygen-carrying protein in the red blood cells).

Anemia reduces the amount of oxygen available to all the cells of the body, so the cells for the body's normal chemical functioning have less available energy. Important processes, such as muscular activity and cell building and repair, slow down and become less efficient. Greater than 95 percent of the body's chemical reactions depend on having optimal oxygen levels in the cells and tissues. As a result, the symptoms of anemia can be very debilitating.

Because the lack of oxygen impairs the body's ability to carry out its numerous chemical reactions, many women with anemia feel extremely tired and fatigued. Because muscular activity is inhibited, they lack endurance and physical stamina. I have had many physically active patients who had to stop pursuing vigorous aerobic exercise programs when they developed anemia, because they lacked the physical energy to continue an active exercise regimen.

When the brain cells lack oxygen, dizziness may result and mental faculties are less sharp. Women who are anemic tend to be pale with poor skin color and tone. They often appear "washed out" and seem listless. They lack the glowing skin color that we tend to associate with good health and vitality. Women with anemia may also suffer from hair loss and brittle, ridged fingernails.

Digestive symptoms include loss of appetite, sore tongue, abdominal pain, heartburn, and diarrhea. In more severe cases, women can suffer from symptoms as varied as headaches, heart palpitations, tingling in the fingers and feet, loss of coordination, and a yellowing of the skin. As you can see, a woman can become quite ill from the physical and mental effects of anemia if her physician does not diagnose her condition properly.

Many cases of anemia are caused by nutritional deficiencies. Without sufficient nutritional factors, the red blood cells cannot grow and mature normally. The most common cause of anemia is iron deficiency. In fact, as many as one-third to one-half of young American women have low or depleted iron stores. The main reason for these low reserves is that women simply don't eat enough iron-rich foods or they lose blood through heavy menstrual bleeding.

Children, adolescents, and women during their reproductive years are at particular risk of iron deficiency anemia. Children and teenage girls need this iron to support growth and development; grown women need it to replace the iron lost in the monthly menstrual period. This increased need for iron persists until menopause, when the monthly blood loss finally ceases. Elderly women are still susceptible to developing anemia because they tend to eat less and have a nutrient-poor diet, especially if they live alone or have a limited income.

Pregnancy and the postpartum period are also vulnerable times for women because fetuses and breast-feeding infants take iron from the mother. Women athletes also have an increased need for iron during training because of the metabolic demands of heavy exercise.

Some women develop iron deficiency anemia because their bodies are unable to absorb and assimilate iron properly. Iron absorption may be decreased by chronic diarrhea, laxative abuse, or malabsorption due to diseases such as celiac disease and sprue. It may also occur due to nutritional deficiencies of vitamins and minerals needed for the health of the digestive tract.

Another common reason for the development of iron deficiency anemia is excessive blood loss. This is commonly seen in women who suffer from heavy or prolonged menstrual bleeding caused by hormonal imbalances that result in fibroid tumors, endometriosis, uterine cancer or other conditions. Women who use intrauterine devices for contraception are also at higher risk of blood loss, as are women who overuse anti-inflammatory medications such as aspirin or ibuprofen, which can cause blood loss through irritation of the digestive tract.

Besides iron, other nutrients are needed for healthy red blood cell growth and maturation. Deficiencies of vitamin B12, folic acid, and vitamin B6 are also common causes of anemia. Vitamin E is important for red blood cell survival. Medical research done on subjects deficient in vitamin E has shown that this nutrient helps prolong the life span of red blood cells.

For many American women, anemia can complicate a pre-existing health-care condition. For example, anemia often accompanies thyroid disease, rheumatoid arthritis, and chronic kidney disease, as well as recurring or chronic infections. Anemia contributes to the fatigue and lack of energy that affect people suffering from these health problems.

Anemia can also be caused by drugs that destroy or interfere with the utilization of the nutrients necessary for the health and maturation of the red blood cells. These drugs include oral contraceptives, alcohol, and anticonvulsive agents such as Dilantin. In all of these cases, the underlying causes of anemia must be reversed and corrected in order to re-establish healthy, normal red blood cells capable of carrying sufficient oxygen. When the anemia is corrected, the accompanying fatigue and lethargy will also be corrected.

In summary, fatigue is an important symptom in many common health problems of women, including neurotransmitter imbalances, ME/CFS, candida infections, allergies, PMS, menopause, weak adrenals, hypothyroidism, anemia, and depression.

Work With a Physician Who Will Properly Diagnose Your Condition

It is important that you work with a physician who will take your complaint of fatigue and tiredness seriously and not simply screen you for the few common conditions that fall within easy, conventional medicine diagnostics, such as anemia and thyroid disease. Don't let a doctor imply that "it's all in your head."

Work with a physician who will take your complaints seriously and will dig deeper to find the cause of your symptoms. Choose a health care provider who will be willing to screen you for conditions like weak adrenal function, candida and allergies that are often overlooked by physicians, if that seems appropriate, given the nature of your fatigue symptoms. Otherwise, your underlying condition will never be treated and your fatigue will continue to be a major problem.

In Chapter 2, I share with you a workbook that I developed that will help you pinpoint any underlying physical problems that may be compounding your fatigue. It will also help you evaluate how your lifestyle habits may be contributing to increased fatigue and tiredness.

Part II:
Evaluating Your Symptoms

2

The Chronic Fatigue Workbook

In this chapter, I provide you with a very useful workbook that will assist you in pinpointing the risk factors in your own life that may be contributing to your chronic fatigue symptoms. Many of these questions are similar to the medical history that I take with patients.

I recommend that you fill out the questionnaires in this workbook. They will help you to become aware of possible risk factors that may be triggering your fatigue and depression symptoms based on your lifestyle habits. They will also help you to pinpoint the link between any health problems that you may have and your fatigue symptoms.

The workbook will show you areas in your life that need attention and modification so that you can receive the greatest benefit from the treatment chapters in this book. You can also share this information with your own doctor or health care provider, thereby providing more complete data when a medical exam is performed. I have personally found it very helpful when my patients share the following charts with me.

This workbook section can help you evaluate many of the factors that contribute to fatigue and tiredness. First, begin to fill out the checklists of symptoms, starting today. They will help you to better understand which symptoms seem to be most relevant for your issues.

It will be helpful to make several copies of the checklists that pertain to you. If you recall your symptoms for the past month, chart these symptoms as well. The checklists will allow you to see which types of symptoms you have, as well as evaluate their severity. This will make it easier for you to select the specific self-care treatments for symptom relief. Then, as you follow the program, you can keep using the checklists to track your progress.

After you have filled out the checklists, look over the risk factor and lifestyle evaluations that follow. They will help you assess specific areas of your life to see which of your habit patterns may be contributing to your symptoms. Your lifestyle habits are probably significantly impacting the symptoms of fatigue and tiredness that you are experiencing.

By filling out the checklists, you can easily recognize your vulnerable areas. I have also included a chapter on how your doctor or caregiver would likely diagnose the causes of your symptoms from the medical standpoint. When you've completed these evaluations, you will be ready to go on to the self-help chapters and begin your self-care treatment program.

Evaluating Your Symptoms

Chronic Fatigue Syndrome/ Myalgic Encephalomyelitis (ME/CFS)

ME/CFS affects over 1 million people in the United States and 17 million people worldwide. For a true diagnosis of ME/CFS, the symptoms must fulfill certain criteria. Women with chronic fatigue must, with their physician's help, rule out any other disease that can mimic ME/CFS symptoms. The fatigue must have lasted at least six months and be severely debilitating. The fatigue must also be accompanied by other characteristic symptoms (at least four of those listed below in addition to fatigue itself).

Check the symptoms that pertain to you.

	Yes	No
Fatigue that has persisted for six months or more and impairs daily activity by at least 50 percent	____	____
Chills and night sweats	____	____
Sore throat, throat infections without pus	____	____
Painful lymph nodes in the neck or armpits	____	____
Unexplained generalized muscle weakness	____	____
Muscle discomfort (myalgia)	____	____
Joint pains without swelling or redness	____	____
Intolerance to light	____	____
Blind spot in the visual field	____	____
Irritability	____	____
Depression	____	____
Sleep disturbance	____	____
Prolonged (more than 24 hours) generalized fatigue following mild to moderate exercise	____	____
Major symptoms developing over a few hours to a few days	____	____
Forgetfulness, confusion, difficulty thinking, inability to concentrate	____	____
Generalized headaches (different from any before this illness)	____	____

Fibromyalgia

Fibromyalgia is a painful condition that affects 2 to 4 percent of the population, or five million people, mostly women. In fact, women are more affected than men by a 9 to 1 ratio. It is considered to be a syndrome with a number of signs and symptoms that occur together but without an identifiable cause. (In contrast, a disease often has a specific, recognizable cause.)The list of symptoms linked to fibromyalgia is long and can vary from woman to woman.

	Yes	No
Chronic muscle pain, muscle spasms, or tightness	___	___
Numbness or tingling in the face, arms, hands, legs, or feet	___	___
Moderate or severe fatigue and decreased energy and stamina	___	___
Insomnia or waking up feeling just as tired as when you went to sleep	___	___
Stiffness upon waking or after staying in one position for too long	___	___
Tension or migraine headaches	___	___
Difficulty in concentrating and performing simple mental tasks, poor memory	___	___
Jaw and facial tenderness	___	___
Urinary urgency or frequency (irritable bladder)	___	___
Abdominal pain, bloating, nausea, and constipation alternating with diarrhea (irritable bowel syndrome)	___	___
Sensitivity to odors, noise, bright lights and cold	___	___
Feeling depressed, anxious or history of post-traumatic stress disorder	___	___
Sensitivity to certain foods or medications	___	___
Reduced tolerance for exercise and muscle pain after exercise	___	___

Depression

Almost 15 million American adults are affected by depression each year, including twice as many women as men. It is estimated that 30 million people suffer from depression during their lifetime. Check the symptoms that fit you. If your symptoms are severe, be sure to consult your physician. You can also follow the useful self-care suggestions in this book for depression and fatigue to help balance your mood.

	Yes	No
Fatigue	___	___
Feeling tearful, sad, "blue"	___	___
Tendency toward isolation, desire to be alone	___	___
Difficulty in concentrating or making decisions	___	___
Poor mental acuity	___	___
Low self-esteem, little self-confidence	___	___
Self-dislike	___	___
Feeling of hopelessness	___	___
Suicidal thoughts and feelings	___	___
Difficulty sleeping	___	___
Overeating	___	___
Loss of appetite	___	___
Loss of sex drive	___	___
Digestive upsets	___	___
Headache	___	___
Backache	___	___

Premenstrual Syndrome (PMS)

The most commonly experienced PMS symptoms are those that affect a woman's emotional well-being and energy level, including premenstrual fatigue. Other common symptoms include food cravings, bloating, headaches, and skin changes. Check the symptoms that pertain to your PMS pattern.

	Yes	No
Nervous tension	_____	_____
Mood swings	_____	_____
Irritability	_____	_____
Anxiety Headache	_____	_____
Craving for sweets	_____	_____
Increased appetite	_____	_____
Pounding heart	_____	_____
Fatigue	_____	_____
Tremulousness	_____	_____
Depression	_____	_____
Forgetfulness	_____	_____
Crying	_____	_____
Sleeplessness	_____	_____
Weight gain	_____	_____
Swelling of extremities	_____	_____
Breast tenderness	_____	_____
Abdominal bloating	_____	_____
Oily skin	_____	_____
Acne	_____	_____

Menopause

During the transition into menopause, women commonly experience many uncomfortable symptoms, including changes in mood and energy level. Many menopausal women have less energy and vitality than during their younger, reproductive years. Some women find that this affects their lifestyle and range of activities. If you have any of the menopausal symptoms listed below, follow the recommendations for relief in the self-help chapters of this book.

	Yes	No
Cessation of menstruation	____	____
Hot flashes	____	____
Night sweats	____	____
Vaginal dryness	____	____
Skin and hair dryness	____	____
Pain during sexual intercourse	____	____
Decrease in sex drive	____	____
Increase in frequency of vaginal infections	____	____
Increase in urinary frequency	____	____
Loss of urine when sneezing or coughing	____	____
Increased frequency of urinary tract infections	____	____
Anxiety, irritability, depression, mood swings	____	____
Fatigue	____	____
Poor mental acuity and concentration	____	____
Insomnia	____	____
Weight gain	____	____
Poor muscle tone	____	____
Increased muscle weakness	____	____
Loss of muscle and bone mass	____	____

Weak Adrenals

The adrenal glands are part of our stress response system. The adrenals are two triangular-shaped organs, about the size of almonds, resting on top of each kidney. The adrenal glands secrete several dozen hormones to help us regulate stresses of all types. Stress can be a response to strong emotional feelings, such as anxiety or depression, or to physical triggers, such as prolonged physical exertion, an allergic reaction, infectious disease, burns, surgery, or an accident. You are likely to have weak adrenals if you have the symptoms listed below. If so, follow the recommendations in the self-care chapters for optimal adrenal health.

	Yes	No
Fatigue and tiredness	____	____
Difficulty handling life stresses – work, financial, family or other issues	____	____
Staying up too late at night and not having enough sleep, feeling tired in the morning	____	____
Too much intense emotional stress - conflicts with friends, family or co-workers that make you	____	____
Feeling burned out/lack of energy even after a long night of sleep	____	____
Blood sugar imbalances, hypoglycemia	____	____
Allergies including food allergies, asthma and other inflammatory conditions	____	____
Female hormonal and menstrual issues, PMS, perimenopause or menopause symptoms	____	____
Autoimmune diseases, like lupus, rheumatoid arthritis, ulcerative colitis or Crohn's disease	____	____
Frequent infections	____	____

Hypothyroidism

Hypothyroidism is a common cause of tiredness in women. It increases with age and is far more common in women than in men (90 percent of the cases occur in women). If you suspect hypothyroidism on the basis of a positive response to the symptoms listed below, consult your physician. This condition can be easily diagnosed by blood testing and treated with thyroid hormone replacement therapy. Follow the recommendations in the self-care chapters for optimal thyroid health.

	Yes	No
Hoarse voice	___	___
Constipation	___	___
Slowness of speech, thought, and movement	___	___
Fatigue	___	___
Intolerance to cold	___	___
Thickening and scaling of skin	___	___
Facial puffiness	___	___
Delay of deep tendon reflexes	___	___
Low dietary iodine	___	___
Axillary (armpit) temperature below 97.8°F	___	___
Elevated cholesterol	___	___

Candida Infections

Many women with a chronic candida problem suffer not only the common symptoms of chronic vaginal discharge and digestive upsets, but also fatigue and lethargy, as well as other symptoms. If candida seems to be your problem, check with your physician for a thorough evaluation. (The self-care suggestions in this book are also useful for the relief and prevention of candida.)

	Yes	No
Fatigue or lethargy	___	___
Depression	___	___
Poor memory, poor concentration	___	___
Persistent or recurrent vaginal discharge, itching, burning	___	___
Recurrent urinary burning, frequency	___	___
Bad breath	___	___
Joint pain or swelling	___	___
Muscle aches or weakness	___	___
Numbness, tingling, burning	___	___
Headache	___	___
Nasal congestion, discharge, itching, postnasal drip	___	___
Skin rashes	___	___
Cough, tightness in chest, wheezing, shortness of breath	___	___
Poor visual activity, frequent tearing or burning of eyes	___	___
Menstrual dysfunction, cramps, premenstrual tension	___	___
Cravings for sugar, bread, or alcoholic beverages	___	___
Abdominal bloating, pain, constipation, diarrhea, intestinal gas, mucus in bowel movements	___	___

Allergies

Women who have food or environmental allergies are often tired and lethargic if frequently exposed to the offending allergens. Allergens may also trigger uncomfortable symptoms in many different body systems.

	Yes	No
Nasal congestion, sneezing, itching, postnasal drip	___	___
Popping or fullness in ears	___	___
Hives; itching, burning, or flushing of skin	___	___
Frequent or urgent urination	___	___
Sleepiness, slowness, sluggishness, dull feeling	___	___
Headaches	___	___
Depression	___	___
Fatigue	___	___
Tension, anxiety, hyperactivity, restlessness, excitability	___	___
Inability to concentrate, difficulty in remembering words or names	___	___
Redness, itching, or swelling of eyes; watery eyes, blurred vision, pain in eyes	___	___
Shortness of breath, wheezing, coughing, tightness or itching in throat	___	___
Heartburn, indigestion, nausea, vomiting, diarrhea, itching or burning of rectum, abdominal pain or cramps	___	___

Anemia and Heavy Menstrual Flow

The most common symptoms of anemia are listed below. In women, anemia is frequently caused by heavy menstrual bleeding and occurs in pregnancy. Check those symptoms that pertain to you. Some women have very few symptoms, while others have symptoms severe enough to affect their ability to function normally. The worse your symptoms, the more important it is to follow the self-help guidelines in this book.

	Yes	No
Fatigue	____	____
Dizziness	____	____
General weakness	____	____
Paleness	____	____
Profuse or extended menstrual bleeding	____	____
Loss of appetite	____	____
Brittle nails	____	____
Abdominal pain	____	____
Sore tongue	____	____
Yellowing of skin	____	____
Tingling in hands and feet	____	____
Loss of coordination	____	____
Diarrhea	____	____

Evaluating Your Lifestyle Habits

The following charts allow you to evaluate the effect that your lifestyle habits have on your fatigue symptoms. Fill out the charts to see which areas of your life need to be modified to improve your energy level.

Eating Habits Checklist

Check the number of times you eat the following foods.

Foods That Increase Symptoms

Foods	Never	1x a Month	1x a Week	>1x a Week
Coffee				
Cow's milk				
Cow's cheese				
Butter				
Chocolate				
Sugar				
Alcohol				
White bread				
White noodles				
White flour				
Pastries				
Added salt				
Bouillon				
Commercial salad dressing				
Catsup				
Black tea				
Soft drinks				
Hot dogs				
Ham				
Bacon				
Beef				
Lamb				
Pork				

Foods That Decrease Symptoms

Foods	Never	1x a Month	1x a Week	>1x a Week
Avocado				
Green Beans				
Beets				
Broccoli				
Brussels sprouts				
Cabbage				
Carrots				
Celery				
Collard greens				
Cucumbers				
Eggplant				
Garlic				
Horseradish				
Kale				
Legumes				
Lettuce				
Mustard greens				
Okra				
Onions				
Parsnips				
Peas				
Potatoes				
Radishes				
Rutabagas				
Spinach				
Squash				
Sweet potatoes				
Tomatoes				
Turnips				
Turnip greens				
Yams				
Brown rice				
Millet				
Barley				
Oatmeal				

Foods	Never	1x a Month	1x a Week	>1x a Week
Buckwheat				
Rye				
Flaxseeds				
Corn				
Pumpkin seeds				
Sesame seeds				
Sunflower seeds				
Raw almonds				
Raw filberts				
Raw pecans				
Raw walnuts				
Apples				
Bananas				
Berries				
Pears				
Seasonal fruits				
Corn oil				
Flax oil				
Olive oil				
Sesame oil				
Safflower oil				
Eggs				
Poultry				
Fish				

Key to Eating Habits

All foods in the shaded area (from coffee through pork) are high-stress foods that are difficult to digest, stress the body's systems, and can increase the symptoms of chronic fatigue and tiredness. If you eat many of these foods, or if you eat any of these foods frequently, your nutritional habits may be contributing significantly to your symptoms.

All foods in the unshaded area (from avocado through fish) are high-nutrient, low-stress foods that can be eaten on a regular basis by women who are recovering from fatigue. If your energy levels are approaching normal, you should include these foods frequently in your diet. Women who are just beginning a chronic fatigue self-help program will need a more restricted eating plan, as discussed in the chapters on diet and meal planning.

For further guidance on food selection, read Chapter 4, 5 and 6 which discuss the foods to avoid and foods to eat as well as helpful menus, meal plans and recipes. These recommendations and programs will help women just beginning a chronic fatigue recovery program as well as those who need a good maintenance plan.

Exercise Habits Checklist

Check the frequency with which you do any of the following:

Activity	Never	1x a Month	1 or 2x a Wk.	3x a Week +
Aerobic exercise				
Bicycling				
Bowling				
Dancing				
Gardening				
Golf				
Ice skating				
Jogging				
Roller skating				
Stretching				
Swimming				
Walking				
Weight lifting (small weights)				

Key to Exercise Habits

Many women with chronic fatigue tend to lack physical endurance and stamina. Even women who are accustomed to an active and vigorous exercise regimen may start to feel that any physical activity at all is just too difficult and may decide to stop exercising completely. This can have negative physiological effects on the body and actually worsen the fatigue symptoms. Although vigorous exercise may tire out a woman suffering from chronic fatigue, gentle exercise provides the benefits of oxygenation, improved blood circulation, and muscle and joint flexibility.

Exercise also helps to improve the mood as well as emotional and mental well-being, a welcome relief to many women with chronic fatigue. Select one of the less strenuous exercises given in the checklist and do it two or three times per week, to begin. I include in this book gentle stretching exercise routines that you may find pleasant and easy to do.

Major Stress Evaluation

Major life stress can have a significant impact on the symptoms of chronic fatigue as well as other health problems. It is helpful to assess your own level of stress to see how it may be impacting your health. One popular tool is the Holmes and Rahe Social Readjustment Rating Scale that was adapted for women and identifies events that cause stress.

Check each stressful event that applies to you. This will help you evaluate the level of major stress in your life.

Life Events

_____ Death of spouse or close family member

_____ Divorce from spouse

_____ Death of a close friend

_____ Legal separation from spouse

_____ Loss of job

_____ Radical loss of financial security

_____ Major personal injury or illness (gynecologic or other cause)

_____ Future surgery for gynecologic or other illness

_____ Beginning a new marriage

_____ Foreclosure of mortgage or loan

_____ Lawsuit lodged against you

_____ Marriage reconciliation

_____ Change in health of a family member

_____ Major trouble with boss or co-workers

_____ Increase in responsibility—job or home

_____ Learning you are pregnant

_____ Difficulties with your sexual abilities

_____ Gaining a new family member

_____ Change to a different job

_____ Increase in number of marital arguments

_____ New loan or mortgage of more than $100,000

_____ Son or daughter leaving home

_____ Major disagreement with in-laws or friends

_____ Recognition for outstanding achievements

_____ Spouse begins or stops work

_____ Begin or end education

_____ Undergo a change in living conditions

_____ Revise or alter your personal habits

_____ Change in work hours or conditions

_____ Change of residence

_____ Change your school or major in school

_____ Alterations in your recreational activities

_____ Change in church or club activities

_____ Change in social activities

_____ Change in sleeping habits

_____ Change in number of family get-togethers

_____ Diet or eating habits are changed

_____ You go on vacation

_____ The year-end holidays occur

_____ You commit a minor violation of the law

Key to Major Stress Evaluation

Checking many items in the first third of this scale indicates major life stress and a possible vulnerability to serious illness. As you go down the list, the stresses decrease in the degree to which they cause major emotional and physical dislocation. For example, a death or divorce is much more traumatic for most people than changing their school or major, if you are a student. In other words, the more items checked in the first third, the higher your stress quotient.

When recovering from fatigue and tiredness, it is important to do everything possible to manage your stress in a healthy way. Eat the foods that provide a high-nutrient/low-stress diet, do gentle exercise on a regular basis, and learn the methods for managing stress given in the chapter on stress reduction and deep breathing.

If you checked fewer items, you are probably at lower risk of illness caused by stress. But because the cumulative effect of stress in life can still play a role in worsening fatigue, you may find that you can benefit from practicing the techniques in the chapters on stress reduction. Stress management is very important in helping you to recover from fatigue, tiredness and depression, whether the underlying cause is physical or emotional.

Daily Stress Evaluation

This evaluation is very important for women with chronic fatigue. Not all stresses have as major impact in our lives, as do death, divorce, or personal injury. Most of us are exposed to a multitude of small life stresses on a daily basis. In filling out this questionnaire, you may find a number of stresses that are worsening fatigue, tiredness and depression in your life.

In addition, the effects of these stresses can be cumulative. They can be a major factor in creating chronic wear and tear on our immune, endocrine and circulatory systems. In addition, daily stress often triggers chronic muscle tension and pain.

Check each item that seems to apply to you.

Work

_____ **Too much responsibility.** You feel you have to push too hard to do your work. There are too many demands made of you. You feel very pressured by all of this responsibility. You worry about getting all your work done and doing it well.

_____ **Time urgency.** You worry about getting your work done on time. You always feel rushed. It feels like there are not enough hours in the day to complete your work.

_____ **Job instability.** You are concerned about losing your job. There are layoffs at your company. There is much insecurity and concern among your fellow employees about their job security.

_____ **Job performance.** You don't feel that you are working up to your maximum capability due to outside pressures or stress. You are unhappy with your job performance and concerned about job security as a result.

_____ **Difficulty getting along with co-workers and boss.** Your boss is too picky and critical. Your boss demands too much. You must work closely with co-workers who are difficult to get along with.

_____ **Understimulation.** Work is boring. The lack of stimulation makes you tired. You wish you were some-where else.

___ **Uncomfortable physical plant.** Lights are too bright or too dim; noises are too loud. You're exposed to noxious fumes or chemicals. There is too much activity going on around you, making it difficult to concentrate.

Spouse or Significant Other

___ **Hostile communication.** There is too much negative emotion and drama. You are always upset and angry. There is not enough peace and quiet.

___ **Not enough communication.** There is not enough discussion of feelings or issues. You both tend to hold in your feelings. You feel that an emotional bond is lacking between you.

___ **Discrepancy in communication.** One person talks about feelings too much, the other person too little.

___ **Affection.** You do not feel you receive enough affection. There is not enough holding, touching, and loving in your relationship. Or, you are made uncomfortable by your partner's demands.

___ **Sexuality.** There is not enough sexual intimacy. You feel deprived by your partner. Or, your partner demands sexual relations too often. You feel pressured.

___ **Children.** They make too much noise. They make too many demands on your time. They are hard to discipline.

___ **Organization.** Home is poorly organized. It always seems messy; chores are half-finished.

___ **Time.** There is too much to do in the home and never enough time to get it all done.

___ **Responsibility.** You need more help. There are too many demands on your time and energy.

Your Emotional State

____ **Too much anxiety.** You worry too much about every little thing. You constantly worry about what can go wrong in your life.

____ **Victimization.** Everyone is taking advantage of you or wants to hurt you.

____ **Poor self-image.** You don't like yourself enough. You are always finding fault with yourself.

____ **Too critical.** You are always finding fault with others. You always look at what is wrong with other people rather than seeing their virtues.

____ **Inability to relax.** You are always wound up. It is difficult for you to relax. You are tense and restless.

____ **Not enough self-renewal.** You don't play enough or take enough time off to relax and have fun. Life isn't fun and enjoyable as a result.

____ **Feeling of depression.** You feel blue, isolated, and tearful. You feel a sense of self-blame and hopelessness. Fatigue and low energy are problems.

____ **Too angry.** Small life issues seem to upset you unduly. You find yourself becoming angry and irritable with your husband, children, or clients.

Key to Daily Stress Evaluation

The effects of these daily stresses are cumulative and can be a major factor in triggering exhaustion. Becoming aware of them is the first step toward lessening their effect on your life. Methods for reducing stresses and helping your body deal with them are given in the chapters of this book on renewing your mind, stress reduction, breathing exercises, stretches and acupressure.

How Stress Affects Your Body

Each woman accumulates stress in a different way, tensing and contracting different sets of muscles in a pattern that is unique to her. Increased tension in your muscles worsens chronic fatigue. Muscle tension cuts off circulation and oxygenation to the affected parts of the body. Waste products of metabolism accumulate. This increase in waste products worsens your level of fatigue and lowers your energy and vitality. This evaluation should help you become aware of where you tend to carry stress.

Check the places where tension most commonly localizes in your body.

_____ Low back Pelvic area
_____ Stomach muscles
_____ Thighs and calves
_____ Chest
_____ Shoulders Arms
_____ Neck and throat
_____ Headache
_____ Grinding teeth
_____ Eyestrain

Key to How Stress Affects Your Body

It is important to be aware of where you store tension. When you feel tension building up in these areas, begin deep breathing exercises or use one of the stress reduction techniques that I share with you in the self-care chapters of this book. These techniques can help release muscle tension rapidly.

In the next chapter, I want to share with you important information on the steps that your doctor or caregiver is likely to take in diagnosing your symptoms of anxiety and panic attacks from the medical point of view.

3

Diagnosis of Chronic Fatigue

It is very important to consult with a physician or other caregiver to have an accurate diagnosis of the causes of your fatigue and tiredness. Even if you choose to follow a totally all natural treatment program like the one that I share with you in this book, it is still important for your symptoms to be properly evaluated. Of primary importance is for your physician or caregiver to determine if your symptoms are physical in origin or if there are emotional and psychological causes for your fatigue and tiredness that need to be corrected.

There are three steps that your physician or caregiver may need to take in order to accurately diagnose chronic fatigue and tiredness. This includes taking a medical history, doing a physical examination and then ordering or performing diagnostic tests to better evaluate your condition. This can include doing a variety of blood, saliva or urine tests that seem to be most appropriate to your set of signs and symptoms.

I am going to describe the process of diagnosing chronic fatigue in some detail so that you can know what to expect once you start this process with your own doctor or caregiver.

Let's look now at each of these steps. If you have not already done so, I recommend that you fill out the workbook section questionnaires on your current diet, stress triggers, exercise habits, patterns of muscle tension and other risk factors.

You may want to share your responses to these questionnaires with your health care provider because they can offer valuable clues to help discover a medical problem that hasn't yet been diagnosed. Also, be sure to let your physician know if you have any previously diagnosed problems such as hypothyroidism that commonly causes fatigue if not treated or if the dosage of thyroid hormone replacement therapy is not sufficient.

Medical History

Your doctor will begin the process of evaluating the cause of fatigue and tiredness by taking a careful medical history. You will probably be asked about your symptoms and how they are affecting your mood and body. There are quite a number of symptoms that have been linked to fatigue. In fact, fatigue is such a common complaint with many illnesses and many lifestyle factors, that narrowing this down can be quite important to making a proper diagnosis Your doctor should ask you about any previously diagnosed health issues such as anemia, thyroid disease, depression, insomnia, PMS, menopause, ME/CFS, kidney, heart and lung disease and even cancer.

Your caregiver should ask you when you first noticed these symptoms. Was the onset of your fatigue sudden or has it been gradually worsening over time. Does sleep and rest help to lessen your fatigue or have no impact? Do you snore at night or stop breathing for short periods of time during sleep? Is your fatigue affected by the change of seasons, worse during the winter months when the days are shorter and sun exposure is greatly reduced?

It is also important to ask about your diet and if the ingestion of certain foods such as alcohol use or caffeine worsens fatigue or if you have unhealthy eating habits. Do you have a history of substance abuse of drugs, alcohol or food? It is important to know if you have been engaging in excessive physical activity such as training for a competition or marathon or if you have a sedentary lifestyle and are not exercising at all or very little.

In addition, it is important to provide any pertinent information about the use of nutritional supplements and medications. Many prescription and over-the-counter medications may worsen fatigue including antidepressants, antihistamines, muscle relaxants and antihypertensive medication.

Hormonal therapies such as birth control pills or hormone replacement therapy (HRT) may also be affecting your symptoms and should be asked about. Your doctor should find out if the symptoms are related to the timing of your menstrual periods or began to occur with the onset of menopause. This can suggest a possible hormonal trigger for your symptoms.

Risk factors such as dietary and nutritional status and level of personal, work and family stress or if other family members also suffer from depression should be evaluated. Does it appear to be linked to any major life changes such as death or divorce as well as job or relationship changes? These essential lifestyle factors can significantly affect your level of fatigue and tiredness. Unfortunately, many of these factors are more likely to be looked at and evaluated by an alternative health practitioner rather than a conventional medical doctor.

Physical Examination

Your doctor should check your blood pressure and pulse rate to see if they are too low. He or she should exam you for enlarged lymph nodes, check your neck and throat as well as listen to your heart and lungs. Your physician will be checking for abnormalities of the heart rate and rhythm as well as the presence of heart murmurs or abnormal heart sounds that may be linked to conditions that could worsen fatigue. The abdomen should be felt to check for enlargement of the liver or fluid accumulation.

The thyroid gland should be checked for enlargement or nodules. A potentially serious condition that can be overlooked or misdiagnosed is hypothyroidism. This is particularly true with women in menopause, if the symptoms are thought to be due simply to stress or the change of life. Physical signs of this condition that can be seen on physical examination include cool, dry skin, hair loss and swelling of the face, arms, hands and legs.

If you have anemia, you may tend to be pale with poor skin color and tone. Women with anemia often appear "washed out" and seem listless. They lack the glowing skin color that we tend to associate with good health and vitality. You may also suffer from hair loss and brittle, ridged fingernails.

Laboratory Testing

Depending on your age, a complete blood count to check for anemia and possible infection, a chemistry panel to check for liver disease, kidney failure or malnutrition, panel, urinalysis, erythrocyte sedimentation rate to check for inflammation, thyroid function tests, and hormone panels may be done when screening for fatigue. Depending on your medical history and physical examination, other tests may be ordered, also.

Your doctor may choose to have testing of your neurotransmitter levels done. Other tests that may be ordered depending on your symptoms can include testing for candida antibodies, allergy testing, testing for adrenal and digestive function and a hormonal panel. If you don't understand any terms or tests used, ask your physician for more information. An informed and educated woman patient can do a much better job planning and participating in her own wellness program. Let's now look at the different types of testing that may be done.

Brain chemistry testing is somewhat controversial. Some physicians believe strongly in the value of this type of testing to assist in the diagnosis of depression and help to select the most effective therapies, especially the amino acids, vitamins and minerals necessary to manufacture neurotransmitters within your body. In contrast, other practitioners think that that these tests are worthless and do not order them. The feelings on this issue can run very strongly from one practitioner to another.

The laboratories that do urine neurotransmitter testing are, in fact, testing the levels of neurotransmitters within the whole body, rather than specifically the brain levels of these chemicals. However, the laboratories that run these tests have correlated the levels of these neurotransmitters with specific psychiatric abnormalities like anxiety or depression.

One laboratory, NeuroScience, Inc., (888-342-7272 or www.neurorelief com) is a leader in the development of neurotransmitter testing. They have developed sensitive testing for these neurochemicals that can be done through your urine. The test is simple to do, non-invasive, and can be done in the privacy of your own home. In addition to NeuroScience, there are many other similar laboratories that offer neurotransmitter testing.

Depression can cause digestive symptoms such as diminished or increased appetite, nausea, diarrhea and constipation. If you have digestive symptoms, your doctor may want to evaluate your digestive function to rule out other causes of these symptoms including bacterial, yeast and parasite infections, allergies to common foods like wheat, milk, soy and eggs, deficient enzyme production within the digestive tract and any signs of intestinal bleeding. This can be readily done with a stool sample that is then sent to the laboratory for analysis.

Testing of adrenal function as a cause of fatigue and tiredness is difficult to diagnose by traditional blood testing. This is because conventional doctors are looking for more extreme states of adrenal failure (Addison's Disease) or hyperactivity. Alternative medical doctors are more likely to do blood, urine and saliva tests to determine less extreme levels of adrenal stress that may be causing your symptoms. Your doctor may test levels of adrenal hormones and chemicals including cortisol, DHEA, norepinephrine and epinephrine that can help to indicate your level of adrenal function.

Conventional physicians usually test for food allergies by doing skin tests and blood testing. Unfortunately, these tests are often inaccurate in determining actual food sensitivities. Many people test positively to many healthy foods that they are not allergic to. Some holistic physicians test for food allergies by doing sublingual provocative tests. In this test, a food extract is placed under the tongue to see whether it elicits a reaction. Neutralizing antidotes are then administered to the patient to reduce or eliminate symptoms. This test, however, is not used by traditional allergists.

Finally, there is a blood test called the ELISA (enzyme-linked immunoabsorbent assey) that measures the amount of allergen-specific antibodies in your blood. The advantage of allergy blood testing is that it requires only one needle stick (unlike skin testing). However, these tests are more expensive and may not be covered by your health insurance.

Candida vaginitis can be diagnosed by a slide in which vaginal discharge is examined under the microscope looking for signs of infection. Candida Antigen and Antibody Panel can be done by taking a blood sample to diagnose the presence of candida in your body. Systemic candida infection is characterized by markedly elevated levels of IgG, IgA, and IgM antibodies.

However, the interpretation of Candida antibody levels is complicated since these antibodies are also detected in 20 to 30 percent of healthy people and the antibody response is blunted in patients whose immune system is compromised. As a result, your doctor will likely order testing for candida antigen detection. Stool testing can also be done to evaluate your level of yeast in the body but is considered less reliable.

The diagnosis of hypothyroidism is confirmed with blood tests that measure the level of your main thyroid hormone, thyroxine, and TSH (thyroid stimulating hormone) produced by the pituitary gland. With this condition, thyroxine levels are too low and your TSH levels are too low. TSH levels are usually elevated in order to send a signal to your thyroid gland to produce more hormones. If these tests are abnormal, your doctor may order the antithyroid antibody test to determine if you have autoimmune thyroiditis or Hashimoto's disease, in which the body's defense system attacks the thyroid gland.

On rare occasions, your doctor may also order a thyroid ultrasound or thyroid scan. With a thyroid scan, a radioactive isotope is injected into the vein inside your elbow or hand. This will help to produce an image of your thyroid gland.

Testing of adrenal function as a cause of anxiety and panic attacks is difficult to diagnose by traditional blood testing. This is because conventional doctors are looking for more extreme states of adrenal failure (Addison's Disease) or hyperactivity. Alternative medical doctors are more likely to do blood, urine and saliva tests to determine less extreme levels of adrenal stress that may be causing your symptoms. Your doctor may want to tests levels of adrenal hormones and chemicals including cortisol,

DHEA, norepinephrine and epinephrine that can help to indicate adrenal function.

If your doctor suspects that either PMS or menopause are the cause of your fatigue and tiredness, he or she may want to order hormone testing. Until the 1990's, the method for checking women's hormone levels had severe limitations. A single blood sample was taken and analyzed, though the results of this one-time check were unhelpful, given the ebb and flow of your hormone levels throughout the month In addition, the stress of having blood drawn was enough to throw off a woman's hormone levels and skew the results.

Fortunately, female hormone testing done through saliva samples are also now commonly available. Saliva testing is not only non-invasive (no needle sticks!), but it is also highly accurate. These tests can help to evaluate your hormonal status and assist in the design of a treatment program individualized for your anxiety symptoms that can deliver the maximum benefits with minimum risk of side effects.

Best of all, saliva hormone testing is accessible. Even physicians who still don't routinely order saliva hormone testing will usually do so if a patient requests it. You can even order a limited saliva hormone test kit on your own directly from a laboratory, without a doctor's prescription.

Like blood, saliva closely mirrors hormone levels in your body's tissues. However, saliva is a particularly accurate indicator of free (unbound) hormone levels. This is the key, as only free hormones are active, meaning that they can affect the hormone-sensitive tissues in your breasts, brain, heart, and uterus. Saliva testing therefore provides a superior measure of the levels of hormones that actually affect vital body systems, mood, tissue levels of sodium and fluid, and many other important functions.

Additionally, blood testing only provides a one-time "snapshot" of hormone levels, whereas saliva testing provides a dynamic picture of hormonal ebb and flow over an entire menstrual cycle. In fact, saliva samples are collected during the month, all at the same time of day, and then sent to a laboratory. The lab measures and charts your progesterone and estradiol (your most prevalent and potent form of estrogen) levels. These results are compared to normal patterns. Finally, saliva testing is easy, stress-free and non-invasive. You can collect your own saliva samples, which means you don't have to go to your doctor's office or a lab. Plus, there's no need to draw blood.

If you think saliva hormone testing is right for you, consider consulting your physician. Having your doctor order the test has two advantages: The profile is more extensive, and your insurance may cover the cost. A number of laboratories perform the test. If your doctor doesn't order the test, or you simply want insight to help you develop your own self-care regimen, you can order a test kit from laboratories through the Internet.

Once a definitive diagnosis of fatigue is made, whether physical or psychological, effective treatment can then be instituted to relieve the symptoms and restore your physical energy, mood and emotional balance. For more details, refer to the treatment sections of this book in which I share my very effective treatment program as well as the most up-to-date information on medical therapies.

Part III:
Finding the Solution

4

The Chronic Fatigue Healing Program

I am thrilled that you are ready to being your treatment program! The self-care chapters of this book will be very helpful in providing you with the relief and healing that you are looking for. I am certain that these healing resources will be as beneficial for you as they have been for so many of my patients as well as myself. In the chapters that follow, you'll find helpful self-care treatments. These include my dietary and nutritional supplements program, menus, meal plans and delicious recipes.

I have included chapters on renewing your mind, breathing meditations, stress reduction, exercise, acupressure points and stretching programs. In doing the exercises or stretches, I recommend that you choose the exercises that are focused on your combination of symptoms.

There are two ways that you can work with the treatment chapters. You can either begin by going to the chapters that most appeal to you and work with those therapies, first. However, I do recommend that you start right away by reading the dietary and nutritional supplement chapters, no matter what other chapters you work with. The chronic fatigue relief diet and the therapeutic nutritional supplement program are essential to successfully eliminate your chronic fatigue and depression symptoms. You can also read straight through the rest of the book, get a general overview of the various approaches, and find those you are interested in trying.

Establish the regimen that works for you and use it each month. Whichever way you choose to approach the treatment chapters, if you follow the program faithfully, you will begin to see great improvements in your symptoms very quickly— often within a month or two. My program will also support your general health and well-being. Many of my patients have been thrilled that they have also enjoyed more energy, vitality, clarity of mind and resistance to illness by following these recommendations.

5

Dietary Principles for Relief of Chronic Fatigue

In this chapter, I would like to share with you much important information about the crucial role that food selection plays in either reducing or intensifying your symptoms of chronic fatigue, tiredness and depression. I have found during my years of practice that if women ignore the importance of nutrition in their anti-fatigue program, they have great difficulty getting entirely well.

Women recovering from fatigue need to follow a low-stress diet that is easy to digest and high in nutritional value. Although food provides the energy to fuel the hundreds of thousands of chemical reactions that occur continuously, some foods are not easily used or well tolerated by the body. In fact, the anti-fatigue diet that I have created for my patients is one of the cornerstones of my self-care program.

Many important studies in the field of diet and nutrition over the past few decades have corroborated that certain foods, beverages and food additives can actually worsen or trigger fatigue and depression in women. All women who suffer from fatigue should eliminate these foods, no matter what the cause of the symptoms. For example, I have found that eliminating foods such as wheat and dairy products can help relieve the symptoms of fibromyalgia.

My own findings were reinforced by a study presented at the annual meeting of the American College of Nutrition. In this study, fibromyalgia patients agreed to avoid wheat, dairy products, sugar, corn, or citrus fruits. After two weeks, an incredible 76 percent of the patients reported a reduction of headaches, fatigue, and abdominal bloating, with nearly half also reporting a significant reduction in their pain. Most telling was the fact that their symptoms returned when these foods were reintroduced into their diet.

Similarly, wheat, dairy products and other common reactive foods can also depress your energy if you suffer from food allergies. Many women with chronic fatigue due, in part to food allergies, often have difficulty digesting and processing these types of foods which can cause an exaggerated immune response. Because allergens such as wheat and dairy products stress your adrenals, repeated allergic reactions can actually weaken the adrenals over time. This greatly increases your susceptibility to stress of all types and can lead to fatigue and low energy.

My patient, Jessica, had symptoms that were typical of this pattern. She suffered for years with chronic fatigue and tiredness, irritable bowel syndrome and headaches. When she was finally diagnosed with multiple food allergies and eliminated wheat, dairy and other offending foods from her diet, her symptoms were significantly diminished and her level of energy was greatly improved.

The importance of diet as a risk factor for chronic fatigue is equally true in chemical, hormonal or emotionally-based cases of fatigue, tiredness and depression. Happily, research studies have also found certain foods to be beneficial for their mood-stabilizing and energizing properties. Thus, your food selection plays an important role in how well you heal from your symptoms and restores your energy and vitality.

In my practice, I have been thrilled by the benefits of the anti-fatigue diet for my patients and how well it relieves needless suffering. I have seen thousands of women struggling with fatigue symptoms, due to many different physical and emotional causes, significantly improve when they changed their diets.

My therapeutic diet is an essential part of the treatment program for fatigue caused by brain chemistry imbalances, fibromyalgia, depression, food allergies, menopause, thyroid disease, infectious diseases as well as other causes. In fact, I have found that continuing to have stressful eating habits even works against other therapeutic measures a patient may institute, such as counseling or the use of antidepressant medication.

In this chapter, I list and discuss in detail the foods that worsen fatigue and depression and should be avoided. The list may surprise you because it contains foods that are considered staples of the American diet. Many women with fatigue unwittingly eat a diet that worsens their symptoms. I also discuss foods that can improve and enhance your emotional well-being as well as your general state of health. This information is based on successfully assisting thousands of patients who suffered from fatigue and noted significant relief of their symptoms when following this program. It is also based on the scientific and medical research in this field.

Foods to Avoid

It is important to eliminate all foods that diminish your energy reserves. These include foods that are difficult to digest, as well as foods that are toxic and damaging to the body.

The process of digestion itself takes a lot of energy. Digestion must occur before the body can extract energy from the foods you eat. Proteins must be broken down into amino acids, complex carbohydrates into simple sugars, and fats into fatty acids. For these breakdowns to occur, food is chemically acted upon by stomach acid, hormones, pancreatic enzymes, and fat emulsifiers, as well as by the mechanical process that propels food through the entire length of the digestive tract. Once the food is broken down, it must then be absorbed from the digestive tract and taken into the blood. From there, the food particles circulate to cells throughout the body. At this cellular level, the energy contained in the food is finally captured to fuel the body's many chemical and physiological reactions.

This entire process requires a great deal of work. The body needs a lot of reserve energy to produce the chemicals involved in the digestive process. As a result, women with chronic fatigue need to eat foods that require the least amount of work to break down, yet still contain the highest level of nutrients.

Unfortunately, many of the most commonly eaten foods in our society are hard to digest. These include foods that are high in saturated fats, sugars, and animal protein. The long list includes pizza, steaks, bacon, cheeseburgers, French fries, doughnuts, ice cream, hot dogs, chocolate and many other processed and high-stress foods.

For example, the body must work hard to digest a meal of a thick steak, French fries, buttered bread, wine, and a chocolate dessert. This meal is laden with saturated fats, red meat protein, and sugar. On finishing this meal, a woman will feel overly full and more tired than before she started eating.

In contrast, a light meal of soup, mixed green salad and fresh fruit slices is full of vitamins, minerals, carbohydrates, and easy to digest vegetable-based protein. It is also low in fat and refined sugar. These foods are much more likely to leave you feeling energized and comfortable.

Other foods stress the body through their toxicity. There are many mechanisms by which a food can increase fatigue. Some foods have a toxic effect that damages the cells and affects their ability to function. One good example is alcohol, which is particularly toxic to the liver, brain, and nervous system.

Some foods, such as alcohol and sugar, promote the growth of pathological organisms like candida, which can worsen fatigue. Many food additives and preservatives like MSG can cause a toxic or allergic reaction in susceptible women. The following foods should be avoided by women with chronic fatigue and depression, either because they are difficult to digest or because of their toxic effects on the body.

Caffeine. Coffee, black tea, soft drinks, and chocolate—all these foods contain caffeine, an unhealthy stimulant used to increase energy levels and alertness and decrease fatigue. Many women with chronic fatigue mistakenly use caffeine as a pick-me-up to help them get through the day's tasks.

Unfortunately, caffeine can actually worsen fatigue. Even small amounts can cause susceptible women to become jittery. After the initial pickup, women with chronic fatigue find that caffeine intake makes them more tired than before. It depletes energy and physical reserves by stressing the nervous system and exhausting the adrenal glands.

Caffeine also depletes the body's stores of B-complex vitamins and essential minerals, which are important in the chemical reactions that convert food to usable energy as well as helping to balance your brain and hormones. Deficiency of these nutrients worsens fatigue.

Depletion of B-complex vitamins interferes with carbohydrate metabolism and healthy liver function, which helps to regulate estrogen levels. An imbalance in estrogen and progesterone can worsen fatigue and mood swings in women with symptoms of PMS or menopause. Many menopausal women also complain that caffeine increases the frequency of hot flashes. Coffee, black tea, chocolate, and soft drinks all act to inhibit iron absorption, thus worsening anemia, a common cause of fatigue and tiredness.

Sugar. Like caffeine, sugar depletes the body's B-complex vitamins and minerals, thereby increasing nervous tension, moodiness and irritability. Excessive glucose intake disrupts carbohydrate metabolism directly by overworking the pancreas and adrenal glands, worsening the symptoms of fatigue and hypoglycemia. Too much sugar also intensifies fatigue by causing vasoconstriction (the narrowing of the diameter of blood vessels) and putting stress on the nervous system. Candida feeds on sugar, so overindulging in this high-stress food worsens chronic candida infections, another common cause of fatigue.

Unfortunately, sugar addiction is common in our society among people of all ages. Many people use sweet foods as a way to deal with their frustrations and other upsets. As a result, most Americans eat too much sugar. In fact, the average American eats 120 pounds per year! Many convenience foods, including salad dressing, ketchup, and relish, contain high levels of both sugar and salt. Sugar is the main ingredient in soft drinks and in desserts such as candies, cookies, cakes, and ice cream. Highly sugared foods also lead to tooth loss through tooth decay and gum disease. Of even greater significance is the fact that excess sugar intake can worsen diabetes.

In summary, sugar stresses many bodily systems, worsens your health, and intensifies fatigue and tiredness. Try to satisfy your sweet tooth instead with healthier foods, such as fresh fruit or grain-based desserts like oatmeal cookies sweetened with healthy sugar substitutes like stevia or xylitol. You will find that small amounts of these foods can satisfy your cravings. Instead of disrupting your mood and energy level, they actually have a healthful and balancing effect.

Alcohol. Women with chronic fatigue should avoid alcohol entirely. Alcohol has a sedative effect. Many women with fatigue caused by PMS, menopause, ME/CFS, candida, or allergies find that their bodies do not tolerate even small amounts of alcohol. Besides worsening fatigue and making women feel sleepy, alcohol affects mental faculties.

Women with chronic fatigue often complain that alcohol makes them feel "spacey," "ungrounded;' and unable to concentrate or process information efficiently. Alcohol also depletes the body's B-complex vitamins and minerals such as magnesium by disrupting carbohydrate metabolism. In women with PMS, depletion of magnesium and B-complex vitamins can also intensify menstrual fatigue, depression and mood swings.

Candida thrives not only on sugar, but also on alcohol—so alcohol promotes their growth in the body. Women with candida-related fatigue need to avoid alcohol entirely. Many women with allergies are sensitive to the yeasts in the alcohol, which worsen their allergic symptoms. Alcohol is toxic to the liver and can affect the liver's ability to metabolize hormones efficiently. Excessive alcohol intake has been associated with lack of ovulation and elevated estrogen levels, which can trigger fibroid growth and heavy bleeding, particularly in women who are in transition into menopause and have a progesterone deficiency.

When used carefully—not exceeding 4 ounces of wine per day, 10 ounces of beer, or 1 ounce of hard liquor—alcohol can have a delightfully relaxing effect in women who have normal energy levels and are not sensitive to the effects of alcohol. It can make us more sociable and enhance the taste of food. For optimal health, however, I recommend that women with chronic fatigue use alcohol only very rarely. Women who are particularly susceptible to the negative effects of alcohol shouldn't drink at all.

If you entertain a great deal and enjoy social drinking, try nonalcoholic beverages. A nonalcoholic cocktail, such as mineral water with a twist of lime or lemon or a dash of bitters, is a good substitute. Non-alcoholic beer and wine can be used for special occasions if you feel that you need a direct substitute for an alcohol-based beverage.

Dairy Products. For women with chronic fatigue, dairy products are high-stress foods. This always surprises women, because dairy products have traditionally been touted as one of the four basic food groups, and many women use them as staples in their diet, eating large amounts of cheese, yogurt, milk, and cottage cheese. Yet dairy products are extremely difficult for the body to digest. They can worsen fatigue because the body must use so much energy to break them down before they can be absorbed, assimilated, and finally utilized.

All parts of dairy products are difficult to digest—the saturated fat and the milk protein called casein that is tough and difficult for the body to break down. Many women are also intolerant of lactose, the milk sugar. As a result, efficient digestion of dairy products requires hydrochloric acids, enzymes, and fat emulsifiers, which a fatigued woman may not produce in sufficient quantities.

Many women are also specifically allergic to dairy products, and dairy products intensify allergy symptoms, in general. Besides fatigue and tiredness, users of dairy products often complain of allergy-based nasal congestion, sinus swelling, and postnasal drip. They can also suffer from digestive problems such as bloating, gas, and bowel changes, which can intensify with menstruation. This intolerance to dairy products can hamper the absorption and assimilation of the calcium they contain. Clinical studies have also shown that dairy products decrease iron absorption in anemic women.

Dairy products have many other unhealthy effects on a woman's body. The amino acid tryptophan in milk has a sedative effect that increases fatigue, a real problem for some women the first day or two of their periods, as well as for women suffering from depression. Menopausal women, who suffer from fatigue caused by the decline in hormonal levels, may also be sensitive to the tryptophan levels in dairy products.

Besides worsening fatigue symptoms, the saturated fats in dairy products put women at higher risk of heart disease and cancer of the breast, uterus, and ovaries. Women on a high-fat diet also tend to accumulate excess weight more easily.

Women who have depended on dairy products for their calcium intake naturally wonder what alternative sources they should use. Women concerned about calcium intake can turn to many other good dietary sources of this essential nutrient, including beans, peas, soybeans, sesame seeds, soup stock made from chicken or fish bones, and green leafy vegetables.

For food preparation, soymilk, potato milk, and nut milk are excellent substitutes. These nondairy milks are readily available at health food stores. You can also use a supplement containing calcium, magnesium, and vitamin D to make sure your intake is sufficient.

Red Meat. Like dairy products, red meat tends to increase fatigue because it is difficult for the body to digest. Because of the extremely tough protein found in red meat, as well as its high content of saturated fats, the body must work hard to breakdown the protein to amino acids and the saturated fats to fatty acids. As a result, many women with chronic fatigue feel exhausted after a heavy meal of red meat. Besides the difficulty of digesting red meat and the energy expended in the process, red meat intake can also worsen fatigue in other ways.

The body uses the fatty acids found in red meat (and dairy products) to produce a group of hormones called the series-2 prostaglandins. These hormones, found in tissues throughout the body, have negative health effects. They cause contraction of muscles and blood vessels and thereby worsen cramps, PMS, high blood pressure, and irritable bowel syndrome. These hormones also put stress on the immune function and trigger inflammation. As a result, they can worsen infections of all types, decrease resistance, and trigger allergy symptoms.

Eating meat with high saturated fat content as a major part of the diet, like eating dairy products, puts women at risk of heart disease, breast cancer, and cancer of the reproductive tract, as well as obesity. Women with chronic fatigue should sharply curtail such consumption. Instead of eating meat, obtain your protein from healthier meat sources like free range poultry or omega-3 fatty acid rich fish like salmon, trout, tuna and mackerel. Fish has the added benefit of containing high levels of essential fatty acids, which improve vitality. Vegetable sources of protein, such as legumes, whole grain, starches, raw seeds and nuts are also excellent for a woman recovering from fatigue.

Wheat and Other Gluten-Containing Grains. Besides red meat and dairy products, gluten-containing grains, like wheat, rye and oats, are also often difficult for women with chronic fatigue and depression to digest and handle.

Many women with chronic fatigue have difficulty digesting wheat. The protein in wheat, called gluten, is highly allergenic and difficult for the body to break down, absorb, and assimilate. No matter what the cause of your chronic fatigue, if the symptoms are severe, you should probably eliminate wheat from your diet, at least in the early stages of recovery.

Women with wheat intolerance are prone to fatigue, depression, bloating, intestinal gas, and bowel changes. Wheat consumption by women who are nutritionally sensitive can worsen symptoms of depression and exhaustion. I have seen wheat worsen fatigue in my PMS patients during the week or two before the onset of menses. Many menopausal women tolerate wheat poorly because their digestive tracts are beginning to show the wear and tear of aging and they don't produce enough enzymes to handle wheat efficiently.

Women with allergies often find that wheat, like dairy products, intensifies nasal and sinus congestion as well as fatigue. I also find that women with poor resistance and a tendency toward infections may need to eliminate wheat to boost their immune function. Since wheat is leavened with yeast, it should be also avoided by women with candida infections.

Oats and rye, which also contain gluten, should be eliminated along with wheat. Gluten-free oats are available in health food stores and some supermarkets. Many allergic and severely fatigued women don't even handle corn well. Although corn does not contain gluten, most women who use it frequently may find that they build up an intolerance during times of fatigue.

I have found over the years that one of the least stressful grain for fatigued women is buckwheat. This is probably because it is not commonly eaten in our society. Also, it is not in the same plant family as wheat and other grains. Women with fatigue may be able to tolerate other gluten-free containing grains like brown rice, millet, quinoa and amaranth.

Salt. Although salt does not specifically worsen chronic fatigue, women should watch their salt intake carefully and avoid excessive intake for optimal health and well-being. While sodium is an essential mineral and is necessary for good health, most Americans eat a diet that is actually too high in sodium.

Unfortunately, most processed foods contain large amounts of salt. Frozen and canned foods are often loaded with salt. In fact, one frozen food entree can contribute as much as one-half teaspoon of salt to your daily intake. Large amounts of salt are also commonly found in the American diet as table salt (sodium chloride), MSG (monosodium glutamate), and a variety of food additives. Fast foods such as hamburgers, hot dogs, french fries, pizza, and tacos are loaded with salt and saturated fats. Common processed foods such as soups, potato chips, cheese, olives, salad dressings, and ketchup (to name only a few) are also very high in salt. To make matters worse, many people use too much salt while cooking and seasoning their meals.

Too much salt in the diet can cause many physical symptoms. It can worsen bloating and fluid retention, thereby contributing to the symptoms of PMS and menstrual cramps. Too much salt intake also worsens high blood pressure and is a risk factor in the development of osteoporosis in menopausal women.

For women of all ages, I recommend eliminating added salt in your meals. For flavor, use seasonings such as garlic, herbs, spices, and lemon juice. Seaweed granules, like kelp, are an excellent and good tasting salt substitute. They are an excellent source of iodine that is important if you suffer from hypothyroidism, a common cause of fatigue in women.

Avoid processed foods that are high in salt, including canned foods, olives, pickles, potato chips, tortilla chips, ketchup, and salad dressings. Learn to read labels and look for the word sodium (salt). If it appears high on the list of ingredients, don't buy the product. Many items in health food stores are labeled "no salt added." Some supermarkets offer "no added salt" foods in their diet or health food sections.

Foods to Avoid with Chronic Fatigue

Coffee	Dairy products
Tea (non-herbal)	Red meat
Chocolate	Fried and fatty foods
Cola drinks	Convenience foods
Sugar	Wheat and other gluten-containing grains
Alcohol	Salt

Foods That Help Relieve Chronic Fatigue

The foods that a fatigued woman eats should leave her feeling as good as, if not better than, she felt before the meal. These foods should also support and accelerate the healing process of the illness that underlies the fatigue. To achieve these goals means initially limiting your diet to low-stress foods. As your fatigue symptoms diminish, you can eat a wider range of foods. I help my patients develop an awareness of how their food selections affect their energy levels. If a particular food lowers your energy level each time you eat it, you should eliminate it.

I have found that certain groups of foods are tolerated, even by women who are severely fatigued. These foods include most vegetables, certain fruits, starches, gluten-free grains, legumes, raw seeds and nuts in small amounts, free range poultry and omega-3 fatty acid rich fish like salmon, tuna, trout and mackerel.

If your digestive function is very weak, you may feel better with meals based on even more easily digestible sources of protein like shakes and smoothies made with vegetarian protein powder and easily digestible oils like flaxseed oil instead of most seeds and nuts. I discuss this more in the next chapter on how to create energy enhancing meals. The bottom line, however, is that women with chronic fatigue need to have an easily digestible, stress-free diet. In this section I discuss in detail the benefits of the high nutrient foods that I recommend for fatigue.

Vegetables. These are outstanding foods for the relief of chronic fatigue. Many vegetables are high in calcium, magnesium, and potassium—important minerals that help improve energy, stamina and vitality. Both magnesium and potassium, used in supplemental form in clinical studies, have been shown to increase energy levels dramatically. For women with chronic fatigue who suffer from tension and anxiety, the essential minerals in vegetables have a relaxant effect, relieving muscular tension and balancing the emotions, too.

Both calcium and magnesium act as natural relaxants, a real benefit for women suffering from fatigue and stress. The potassium content of vegetables helps relieve the congestive symptoms of PMS by reducing fluid retention and bloating. Some of the best sources for these minerals include Swiss chard, spinach, broccoli, beet greens, mustard greens, and kale. These vegetables are also high in iron, which can help relieve anemia and menstrual cramps.

Many vegetables are also high in vitamin C, which helps increase capillary permeability and facilitate the flow of essential nutrients throughout the body, as well as the flow of waste products out. This helps to maintain a high level of energy. Vitamin C is also an important anti-stress vitamin because it is needed for healthy adrenal hormone production (the adrenal glands help us maintain a high level of energy and deal with stress).

This is particularly important for women with chronic fatigue caused by infections, allergies, emotional upset, or stress from other origins. Vitamin C is also important for immune function and wound healing. Its anti-infectious properties may help reduce the tendency toward respiratory, bladder, and vaginal infections. Vegetables high in vitamin C include Brussels sprouts, broccoli, cauliflower, kale, red bell peppers, green peppers, parsley, peas, tomatoes, and potatoes.

Vitamin A is important for women with chronic fatigue whose resistance is low and who are thus prone to infections. Vitamin A strengthens the cell walls and protects the mucous membranes. This helps protect you from respiratory disease as well as allergic episodes. Vitamin A deficiency has been linked to fatigue as well as night blindness, skin aging, loss of smell, loss of appetite, and softening of bones and teeth. Luckily, it is easy to get an abundance of vitamin A in the diet from vegetables. Carrots, pumpkin, sweet potatoes, spinach, winter squash, turnip greens, collards, parsley, green onions, and kale are among the vegetables highest in vitamin A.

Vegetables are composed primarily of water and carbohydrates. Because they contain very little protein and fat, they tend to be easy to digest. However, in the early stages of recovery, women with chronic fatigue may find that they more easily digest cooked vegetables. Cooking serves to break down the fiber in the vegetables and render it softer in texture, making less work for the body in the digestion process.

Steaming is the best cooking method, because it preserves the essential nutrients. Some women with extreme fatigue may even want to purée their vegetables in a blender. As you begin to recover your energy, I recommend adding raw foods such as salads, juices, and raw vegetables to your meals for more texture and variety.

Fruits. Fruits also contain a wide range of nutrients that can relieve chronic fatigue. Like many vegetables, fruits are an excellent source of vitamin C, which is important for healthy blood vessels and blood circulation throughout the body, as well as for its anti-stress and immune stimulant properties. Almost all fruits contain some vitamin C, the best sources being citrus fruits like oranges and tangerines, kiwi fruit, currants, strawberries, raspberries, blackberries, peaches, persimmons and papayas. Fruits like oranges, lemons and tangerines are also good sources of bioflavonoids, another essential nutrient that affects blood vessel strength and permeability.

Bioflavonoids also have an anti-inflammatory effect, important to women with allergies, menstrual cramps, or arthritis. Bioflavonoids are supportive of the female reproductive tract and can improve mood and increase energy levels in women with PMS or menopausal symptoms. Although citrus fruits (oranges, grapefruits) are excellent sources of bioflavonoids and vitamin C, they are highly acidic and difficult for many women with chronic fatigue to digest; therefore, such women should avoid them in the early stages of treatment.

Cantaloupes, apricots, papayas, avocados, peaches, persimmons and mangoes are all good sources of immune enhancing vitamin A. Vitamin A is important if your resistance is low and are prone to infections. Vitamin A strengthens the cell walls and protects the mucous membranes. This helps protect you from respiratory disease as well as allergic episodes.

Calcium, magnesium and potassium are important minerals that help improve energy, stamina and vitality. If you suffer from chronic tension and anxiety along with fatigue, calcium and magnesium are helpful because they also have a relaxant effect on the emotions and relieve muscular tension. The best fruit sources of magnesium include avocados, bananas, pineapple juice and grapefruit juice while blackberries, black currants, boysenberries, oranges, raisins, prunes and tangerine juice are your best sources of calcium.

Most fruits are excellent sources of potassium. Particularly good are bananas, orange and grapefruit juice, raisins, prunes, avocados, apricots, figs, currants and cantaloupes.

Eat fruits whole to benefit from their high fiber content, which helps prevent constipation and other digestive irregularities. For snacks and desserts, fresh fruits are excellent substitutes for cookies, candies, cakes, and other foods high in refined sugar that deplete your energy and stress your adrenal glands.

Although fruit is high in sugar, its high fiber content helps slow down absorption of the sugar into the blood circulation and thereby helps stabilize the blood sugar level. I recommend, however, that women with chronic fatigue do not consume fruit juices. Fruit juice does not contain the bulk or fiber of the whole fruit. As a result, it acts more like table sugar and can destabilize your blood sugar level dramatically when used to excess. This can exacerbate fatigue and mood swings.

Starches. Potatoes, sweet potatoes, and yams are soft, well-tolerated carbohydrates that provide an additional source of easy-to-digest protein for women with chronic fatigue. However, they must be combined with other protein containing foods in order to meet your daily protein needs. One of their great benefits, however, is their easy digestibility. You can steam, mash, bake, and eat them alone, or include them in other low-stress dishes and casseroles. Starches combine very well with a variety of vegetables and can form the basis of delicious, low-stress meals. You can also combine them with lentils or split peas in soup.

Potatoes, especially sweet potatoes, are an exceptional source of vitamin A, so they can help boost resistance in women prone to infections and allergies. Potatoes and yams are also good sources of vitamin C and several of the B vitamins that reduce fatigue and help women handle stress better.

Legumes. Beans and peas are excellent sources of energy-building calcium, magnesium, and potassium. I highly recommend their use in a diet to heal fatigue. However, because they also contain high levels of protein, women with severe fatigue may find them difficult to digest at first. For easier digestibility, I recommend beginning with green beans, green peas, split peas, lentils, lima beans, fresh sprouts, and possibly tofu (if you handle soy products well). As your energy level improves, add such delicious legumes as black beans, pinto beans, kidney beans, and chickpeas.

These foods are high in iron and tend to be good sources of copper and zinc. Legumes are very high in vitamin B-complex and vitamin B6, necessary nutrients for the relief and prevention of menstrual fatigue and cramps. They are also excellent sources of protein and, when eaten with grains, provide all the essential amino acids. (Good examples of low-stress grain and legume combinations include meals of beans and buckwheat, or corn bread and split pea soup.) Soy has the additional benefit of being a rich source of phytoestrogens, which can act as virtual mood elevators and have an energizing effect in menopausal women.

Legumes are an excellent source of fiber that can help normalize bowel function. They digest slowly and can help to regulate the blood sugar level, a trait they share with whole grains. As a result, legumes are an excellent food for women with diabetes or blood sugar imbalances. Some women find that gas is a problem when they eat beans. You can minimize gas by taking digestive enzymes and eating beans in small quantities.

Whole Grains. Although you should eliminate wheat and other gluten-containing grains like rye and oats that can stress your immune system and trigger allergies, you may be able to use other grains and grasses like brown rice, millet, buckwheat, quinoa and amaranth. These alternative grains are used to make a wide variety of breads, muffins, bagels, pastas, cereals and flours for baking that are readily available in most health food stores and even some supermarkets. Gluten-free oats are also available in health food stores like Whole Foods Market. You may find that these grain options don't cause the fatigue symptoms that commonly used gluten-containing grains like wheat, oats, and rye often trigger.

Raw Seeds and Nuts. Seeds and nuts are the best sources of the two essential fatty acids, linoleic acid and alpha-linolenic acid. These fatty acids provide the raw materials your body needs to produce the beneficial prostaglandin hormones. Adequate levels of essential fatty acids in your diet are very important in preventing symptoms of PMS, menopause, emotional upsets, allergies, and lowered resistance. The best sources of both fatty acids are raw flax and chia seeds. Other seeds, such as sesame and sunflower seeds, are excellent sources of linoleic acid alone. Seeds and nuts are also excellent sources of the B-complex vitamins and vitamin E, both of which are important anti-stress factors for women with fatigue. These nutrients also help regulate hormonal balance and relieve PMS and menopausal symptoms.

Like vegetables, seeds and nuts are very high in the essential minerals such as magnesium, calcium, and potassium needed by women with fatigue. Particularly beneficial are sesame seeds, sunflower seeds, pistachios, pecans, and almonds. However, they are very high in calories and can be difficult to digest. Therefore, seeds and nuts should be eaten only in small amounts or avoided entirely by women with severe fatigue until their symptoms begin to improve.

Women with fatigue may find, however, that they can tolerate fresh flaxseed oil and their symptoms may even improve with its continued dietary use. Flaxseed oil is one of the best sources of the essential fatty acids needed for production of the beneficial prostaglandin hormones.

The oils in seeds and nuts are very perishable, so avoid exposing them to light, heat, and oxygen. Try to eat them raw, and shell them yourself. Eating them raw and unsalted gives you the benefit of their essential fatty acids (beneficial for skin and hair) and you'll also avoid the negative effects of too much salt. If you buy them already shelled, refrigerate them so their oils don't become rancid. Seeds and nuts make a wonderful garnish on salads, vegetable dishes, and casseroles. As your energy level improves, you can also eat them as a main source of protein with snacks and light meals.

Poultry and Fish. I generally recommend eating meat only in moderation. Particularly good are omega 3 fatty acid-containing fish like salmon, tuna, trout, halibut and mackerel. Fish should be eaten no more than once or twice a week due to the high mercury content in most fish. Also good are free range poultry and game meat. Fatty cuts of red meats like beef, pork, and lamb, contain saturated fats and hard to digest protein.

If you do want to eat meat, your best choice is fish. Unlike other meat, fish contains omega-3 fatty acids that help to reduce fatigue and depression, eliminate inflammation and relax tense muscles. Fish is also an excellent source of minerals, especially iodine and potassium.

If you feel your best using meat as a major source of protein in your anti-fatigue program, I recommend using it in moderate amounts (6 ounces or less per day). Most Americans eat much more protein than is healthy. Excessive amounts of protein are difficult to digest and stress the kidneys. All meats, except fish, are prime sources of unhealthy saturated fats, which put you at higher risk of heart disease and cancer. It is also good to break down the meat fiber in the cooking process by using it in soups, such as chicken and turkey soup, and crockpot or slow cooking which help to make the meat softer, more tender and easy to digest.

I also recommend increasing your intake of other protein sources such as whole grains, beans, raw seeds, and nuts, which contain not only protein but also many other important nutrients. I also recommend buying the meat of organic, free range animals, as their exposure to pesticides, antibiotics, and hormones has been reduced. If you find meat difficult to digest, you may be deficient in hydrochloric acid. Try taking a small amount of hydrochloric acid with every meat-containing meal to see if your digestion improves.

How to Transition to a Healthier Diet

Please don't feel that you need to make all your dietary changes at once. To do so is stressful for anyone, and particularly for a woman with chronic fatigue. Make all nutritional changes gradually and at a pace that feels comfortable to you. Some of my patients eliminate all high stress foods immediately, while others do it slowly over time. You may want to start by eliminating one or two high-stress foods from your diet. After you become comfortable with these initial changes, review the lists of foods to eliminate and foods to emphasize in your diet. Then choose several more foods that you are willing to drop from your menus and try several new ones.

Occasionally, women find that they actually feel worse when they first eliminate high-stress foods such as chocolate, alcohol, coffee, or sugar. This reaction can last a few days or up to several weeks. You may feel irritable, jittery, and suffer from headaches or nasal congestion. You may also crave the foods that you've eliminated. Generally, these are symptoms of withdrawal from foods to which you've actually been addicted. Once the critical period passes, you will begin to feel much better. I generally recommend that women follow the elimination diet carefully throughout their entire recovery from fatigue. In the next two chapters you will find meal plans and recipes to make the process easier.

Once you have regained your energy, I would caution you to continue your avoidance of high stress foods and never eat these foods to excess. Chocolate, alcohol, sugar, colas, coffee, dairy products, and red meat are foods that should be limited in anyone's diet for optimal health and well-being. As long as you follow the general principles proposed in this chapter, your diet should help you recover and maintain your energy and vitality.

6

The Anti-Fatigue Diet – Step 1: Smoothies, Soups & Blenderized Meals

Meal planning is particularly important for women with chronic fatigue. When your energy reserves are low, even the occasional rich meal laden with fats and sugar, eaten at a restaurant or a party, can exhaust you. Frequent meals of high-stress foods can worsen your symptoms significantly and retard your recovery. Women with chronic fatigue need meals high in nutrient content, yet easy to digest. In addition, meals should be quick and easy to prepare, so that food preparation doesn't exhaust your limited energy reserves.

To achieve these goals, you need to follow an elimination diet that features the beneficial foods discussed in the last chapter. High-stress foods, such as alcohol, sugar, chocolate, dairy products, red meats, wheat, and convenience foods, should be strictly eliminated from any good anti-fatigue nutritional program. It is very important to follow these principles very carefully during your recovery from chronic fatigue. The goal is to eat foods that do not worsen your fatigue and that can improve your energy level.

This careful attention to what you eat will pay real dividends as you begin to regain your normal level of energy. My anti-fatigue diet has greatly benefitted many of my patients who were suffering from chronic fatigue. Particularly in the early stages of recovery, women feel better when they follow these diet principles—and notably worse if they go back to eating more stressful foods.

The next two chapters contain helpful information, menus and recipes for the anti-fatigue diet. To make the program easier to use, I have divided the meal plans and recipes into a two-step program. The first step is the most restrictive, intended for women with severe fatigue. The meals in this step are primarily vegetarian based. Easy to digest forms of protein and essential fatty acids like vegetarian protein powder and flax oil have been used in certain recipes. Rather than eating large cuts of meat, such as steaks and burgers which can be difficult to digest, I recommend combining meat with vegetables and whole grains in soups, slow cooked dishes and even pureed to help break down the more difficult to digest meat protein.

If your chronic fatigue is not too severe and you can handle the more broad based, high nutrient diet of stage two, then you can skip this chapter, if you choose, and go on to the next one which contains many delicious meal plans and recipes to help restore your energy, while still eliminating high stress ingredients.

In the second step, intended for women who are starting to feel better, I have expanded the range of foods by adding some fish dishes, a wider variety of grains, and raw foods such as salads. You can also combine these with foods from Step 1. Women with less severe fatigue may want to mix some of the Step 2 dishes with the Step 1 foods right at the beginning.

Remember that how you feel after eating a meal is the ultimate test of how you are handling foods. You must become your own feedback system to evaluate whether the foods you have selected are helping to relieve your fatigue and elevate your vitality and well-being.

I have found that no one diet fits the needs of all different body types. Because of this I have included menus and delicious recipes for women who prefer a vegetarian emphasis, high complex carbohydrate diet as well as dishes and entrees for women who feel their best on a high protein meat-based diet. All of these meal plans and recipes contain ingredients most suitable for providing relief for women suffering from chronic fatigue, tiredness and depression. In addition, the high stress ingredients that can worsen your symptoms have been eliminated.

Let's turn to Step 1 and look at how best to fashion your meals during the early stages when your chronic fatigue, tiredness and depression are the most debilitating. As I mentioned in the previous chapter, the process of digestion itself takes a lot of energy. Digestion must occur before the body can extract energy from the foods you eat. Proteins must be broken down into amino acids, complex carbohydrates into simple sugars, and fats into fatty acids.

For these breakdowns to occur, food is chemically acted upon by stomach acid, hormones, pancreatic enzymes, and fat emulsifiers, as well as by the mechanical process that propels food through the entire length of the digestive tract. Once the food is broken down, it must then be absorbed from the digestive tract and taken into the blood. From there, the food particles circulate to cells throughout the body. At this cellular level, the energy contained in the food is finally captured to fuel the body's many chemical and physiological reactions.

This entire process requires a great deal of work. The body needs a lot of reserve energy to produce the chemicals involved in the digestive process. As a result, women with chronic fatigue need to eat foods that require the least amount of work to break down, yet still contain the highest level of nutrients.

One way to reduce the digestive workload on the body and still be able to extract and absorb the highest amount of essential nutrients is to drink liquid meals: shakes, smoothies, soups, instant whole grain cereals and blenderized meals and pureed foods. Liquefied foods are partially predigested because the ingredients are broken down in the cooking or blenderizing process. This is why I also recommend, eating some cooked foods instead of a completely raw food diet in the early stages of recovery.

Cooking serves to break down the fiber in vegetables, meats, grains and legumes and render them softer in texture, making less work for the body in the digestion process. Steaming is the best cooking method, because it preserves the essential nutrients. Some women with extreme fatigue may even want to purée their vegetables in a blender. As you begin to recover your energy, I recommend adding raw foods such as salads and raw vegetables to your meals for more texture and variety.

Prepackaged Meals

In the initial stages of healing from severe chronic fatigue and tiredness, some of my patients needed to do the least amount of food preparation and cooking and eat only the most easy to digest foods. I've had patients who were so tired initially that all they wanted to do was open a cup of nondairy yogurt or add water to whole grain instant cereal for breakfast.

For dinner, they would open up a can of high quality soup, like organic chicken and rice or vegetable soup or an organic frozen meal, heat the food up and eat. They found this to be a necessary survival strategy. Using premade foods can be helpful when chronic fatigue symptoms are still severe since the fewer the steps between the food preparation and the actual meal, the easier it is to manage, at least in the short run.

However, if you take this route at the beginning of your healing program, there are a few principles that are important to follow.

I recommend buying prepackaged food that comes from organic sources and is labeled as such and that contain high quality, nutrient rich ingredients. For example, choose organic, low salt soups that contain no additives over commercial brands, if at all possible.

It is important to avoid processed foods that are low in essential nutrients and contains ingredients like sugar, white flour and additives that will actually deplete your energy and worsen your fatigue.

In other words, you need to be selective about the quality of any prepackaged foods that you purchase when restoring every little bit of your energy is vital and precious to you. Health food stores tend to have a wider variety of these types of foods so I recommend shopping there instead of your large commercial supermarkets (unless they are well stocked with health food store quality brands).

Besides buying premade canned and packaged high quality foods, you can also make very simple and easy to digest foods at home that are in a liquid base like homemade soups, crockpot and slow cooked meals, smoothies as well as pureed and blenderized meals.

Shakes and Smoothies

Some women find juicing to be beneficial when recovering from fatigue, although you need to be careful to juice mainly vegetables and not drink too much fruit juice. Fruit juice is basically fruit sugar and water with much of the fiber, pulp and other solids removed. The fruit sugar, by itself, without the solids can actually worsen fatigue and adrenal and pancreatic stress.

In contrast, combining whole fruits with other ingredients like rice milk, ground flaxseed and protein powder in a blender for smoothies is much more beneficial since you have the fiber, pulp and even the seeds of the fruit included in the drink. It also provides you with a predigested, high nutrient content complete meal.

Even using fruit juices when they are mixed with protein and oils (like protein powder or ground flaxseed), as is sometimes done with smoothies, is less stressful to the body. This is because the sugar from the juice is absorbed much more slowly and does not cause a hypoglycemic type of effect.

Not only do smoothies and shakes that are partially predigested, liquefied and softened require much less work for your digestive tract to do, but these drinks are absorbed and assimilated very easily, with minimal symptoms of incomplete or poor digestion. They are not as likely to cause symptoms such as bloating, gas and constipation from food remaining in the digestive tract for long periods of time. The essential nutrients from these drinks are much more readily available since they are taken into the body in a liquefied form.

Examples of ingredients that can be used to great benefit in smoothies and shakes when recovering from fatigue include:

Non-dairy milk: rice, almond, soy, flaxseed, coconut, hempseed, and sunflower seed.

Unsweetened nondairy yogurt: Soy, coconut and almond.

Raw seeds and nuts (use in small amounts, if tolerated): Ground flaxseed, chia seeds, hempseeds, sunflowers seeds, pumpkin seeds, almonds, hazelnuts, cashews, pistachios, walnuts and pecans.

Fruit: Bananas, apples, pears, peaches, apricots, papayas, mangos, strawberries, cherries, raspberries, blueberries, boysenberries, watermelon, cantaloupe, acai and other high antioxidant "superfruits".

Protein powder: Rice, soy, legume, mixed source vegan and egg.

Green foods: Spirulina, wild blue-green algae, chlorella, barley greens and wheat grass.

Other: Aloe Vera juice, Coconut water

Blenderized Meals

Let's look at the benefits of blenderized meals since shakes, smoothies, purees and even soups can be prepared in this manner. Processing ingredients in a blender liquefies food, breaking all of its ingredients into extremely small particles, and enhances (or replaces) the mechanical digestive step of chewing. The surface area of the food is dramatically increased, thereby eliminating one of the functions of pancreatic and other enzymes in the breakdown process and therefore requiring less enzyme production. This takes an enormous amount of stress off of the pancreas and other digestive organs.

Foods such as vegetables, fruits, seeds, and nuts can be blenderized to make delicious shakes and drinks. Vegetables such as squash, turnips, yams, sweet potatoes, and potatoes can all be blenderized into purees. Thickened soups that are full of solids like beans and pieces of vegetables can be pureed and made easier to digest. The ingredients can either be raw or precooked by steaming or other stovetop cooking.

Women with chronic fatigue who have very weak digestive systems should consider blenderizing one to two meals per day, with the third meal consisting of easily digestible solid food such as cooked salads, steamed vegetables, cooked grains, and meats like salmon or trout. Fish tends to be softer and easier to digest than tougher, fibrous meats like grilled steak. I have found that very weak or sick patients who substitute one or two blenderized meals per day have much more rapid healing and recovery times from chronic fatigue.

Blenderized drinks can be made from ingredients that are both enzyme-rich and more alkaline because of their high mineral content. Millions of Americans have both low digestive enzyme production and a tendency towards being overly acidic. Drinks such as these can provide therapeutic benefits for both conditions. Liquefying the solid ingredients into a drink further reduces the workload of the pancreas and other digestive organs. These liquid meals can be tremendously beneficial for conditions related to either overacidity or low enzyme production such as fatigue, brain fog, depression, inflammatory conditions, autoimmune problems and even cancer.

Any commercially available blender or food processor can be used. However, I have found that the Vitamix® (vitamix.com) is a power-ful blender that can pulverize virtually any whole food into a liquid (in contrast, juicers tend to extract the juice while discarding the nutrient-rich pulp). This blender can emulsify raw or cooked foods and can be used for any combination of fruits, vegetables, seeds, nuts, liquids, oils or even meat.

Even athletes and others who require very high energy levels to perform in stressful or physically demanding jobs would benefit from relying on at least one blenderized meal per day during times of stress. Over the years, I have developed a number of drink recipes that provide carbohydrates, protein, and fats in an easily digestible form that can replace an entire solid meal. I have included several of these recipes in this chapter. Use these recipes exactly as stated or modify them to your own tastes or specific food tolerances.

Soups and Crock Pot (Slow Cooking) Dishes

There are tremendous benefits from eating soup and crockpot meals when trying to recover from chronic fatigue. With both of these types of meals, fresh, highly nutritious ingredients can be combined. The ingredients are usually cooked at medium or lower temperatures for a longer period of time, thus ensuring that they are extremely tender and easy to digest.

With a covered soup pot or crockpot, there is little evaporation and the food remains in a liquid state that is very rich in essential minerals, protein, carbohydrate, fiber and other important nutrients needed for healing. Preparing these foods is also much easier and less time consuming, once the cooking process has begun. Just turn down the heat and these dishes will cook themselves. Foods cooked in this manner often are very tasty and delicious since the flavors are distributed throughout the entire dish. Other benefits of soups and crockpot cooking is that it gives you flexibility about when to eat your meals and reduces the number of pots, pans and utensils that have to be cleaned and washed.

In contrast, meat on the grill or stovetop needs to be frequently attended to or it will char or dry out from too much cooking. Cooking rice, tomato sauce and other foods on the stovetop also requires constant attention or sticking and burning will occur at the bottom of the pan. Similarly, bread or cookies baking in the oven needs to be monitored and removed in time so that they are not underdone or blackened on the bottom. Unlike soups and crockpot cooking, much food preparation can require a lot of work if you are suffering from fatigue and tiredness.

In the second part of this chapter, I want to share with you some delicious and very nutritious fruit and vegetable drinks as well as a few purees dishes as examples of liquefied, blenderized food preparation. You can enjoy these recipes or create ones of your own! I do want to mention that a wide range of excellent pureed soups, vegetables like butternut squash, sweet potatoes, pumpkin, bean dips and other pureed foods are also readily available in most health food stores. You can purchase these foods for their easy digestability and as a a short cut if you prefer buying premade foods rather than doing a lot of food preparation at home.

Fruit Drinks

All of the ingredients in the following recipes are readily available in health food stores, gourmet markets, and most supermarkets. I strongly recommend using organic ingredients whenever possible, since their nutrient content is higher than that of commercial-grade food. Although these delicious blenderized drinks can be used at any time of the day, many people prefer to have one for breakfast as these drinks can be made quickly and easily consumed.

Raspberry Yogurt Smoothie   Serves 2

¼ cup nondairy yogurt
1 cup raspberries – fresh or frozen
1 banana
¾ cup rice milk
2 teaspoons nondairy protein powder
Sprinkle of Truvia (if desired)

Combine all ingredients in a blender. Puree until smooth and serve.

Blueberry and Greens Shake   Serves 2

This drink is a powerhouse of nutrients! The chlorella and spirulina are powerful green foods that can help replenish your energy. They are both readily available in health food stores or through the Internet.

1 cup nondairy milk
¾ cup blueberries – fresh or frozen
2 tablespoons nondairy protein powder
½ teaspoon chlorella
½ teaspoon spirulina
Sprinkle of Truvia (optional)

In a blender puree the nondairy milk and blueberries. Add the rest of the ingredients and blend well.

Delicious Green Drink   Serves 1

½ cup Concord grape juice
¼ cup water
1 tablespoon ground flaxseed
½ teaspoon chlorella powder
½ teaspoon spirulina powder

Combine all the ingredients together and puree in a blender.

Pomegranate Strawberry Smoothie   Serves 2

This delicious smoothie is rich in essential nutrients that help to restore energy including potassium and vitamin C.

½ cup coconut water
½ cup pomegranate juice
1 cup strawberries – fresh or frozen
1 heaping tablespoon coconut flour
1 banana, sliced

Combine all ingredients in a blender. Puree until smooth and serve.

Blueberry Pomegranate Smoothie   Serves 2

¼ cup nondairy yogurt, unsweetened
¾ cup pomegranate juice
1 cup blueberries, fresh or frozen
1 tablespoon ground flaxseed
1 banana

Combine all ingredients in a blender. Puree until smooth and serve.

Simple Flax Smoothie   **Serves 2**

Flaxseed is not only a tasty addition to smoothies, but it is also nutritious. It is high in essential fatty acids, potassium, magnesium, and calcium.

1 cup vanilla nondairy milk
2 tablespoons ground flaxseed
1 banana

Combine all ingredients in a blender. Blend until smooth and serve.

Peachy Flax Smoothie   **Serves 2**

½ cup orange juice
½ cup unsweetened rice milk
1 cup peaches – fresh or frozen
1 tablespoon rice protein powder
2 teaspoons ground flaxseed
1 banana, sliced

Combine all ingredients in a blender. Puree until smooth and serve.

If using frozen peaches, chopping the peaches beforehand will reduce the puree time in the blender.

Vegetable Drinks

These vegetable drinks are enzyme-rich "liquid salads," made with fresh vegetables and spring water combined in a blender or food processor that is capable of completely liquefying vegetables, such as a VitaMix. The vegetables should be cut up into large pieces before putting them in the food processor. (If you do not have such a powerful food processor, peel vegetables as directed. If you do, the peels can stay on if you like.)

I have also included several recipes to give you some examples of pureed dishes that you can try at home. As mentioned earlier, excellent pureed soups, vegetables like butternut squash, sweet potatoes, pumpkin, bean dips and other foods are also readily available in most health food stores.

If you suffer from overacidity or any inflammatory conditions, be sure to avoid adding hot, spicy, or acidic seasonings and flavorings. Condiments such as chili pepper, Tabasco sauce, black pepper, vinegar, citrus juices, Bloody Mary mix, and Worcestershire sauce can trigger symptoms of overacidity or inflammation in a woman suffering from chronic fatigue and weak digestive function. Many herbs, however, like dill and basil can be safely used as flavoring agents.

Like blenderized drinks, pureed dishes and meals are especially helpful if you have weak digestive function or are recovering from a serious health problem and feel weak and debilitated. People who are frail, thin or elderly may also do well on pureed foods. However, while blenderized drinks are made from raw ingredients, pureed foods are usually cooked before being processed in a blender or food processor.

While these are cooked foods and their enzymes have been deactivated, serving them in pureed form will significantly reduce stress on the digestive process, especially the pancreas. They are easy to digest and help restore strength and vitality during the early healing phase from more serious illness and even chronic fatigue.

Liver Cleanser
Makes 1 cup

6-8 carrots
1 cup dandelion greens
1 cup kale
½ lemon, peeled

Juice the carrots, dandelion greens, kale and lemon. Serve immediately.

Note: Dandelion root is delicious and healthy but also strong in flavor, a little goes a long way.

Vegetable Drink No. 1
Serves 1

¼ cucumber, peeled
1 to 2 tablespoons olive oil
2 to 4 peeled garlic cloves
1 teaspoon maple syrup or rice bran syrup
10 to 12 sprigs parsley
¼ large red bell pepper, seeded
½ teaspoon Bragg Liquid Aminos
½ cooked beet, outer layer scrubbed off
2 cups spring or filtered water
½ carrot, peeled
4 or 5 ice cubes

Combine all the ingredients in a blender or food processor and run it on high speed for 60 to 90 seconds or until the drink is totally liquefied. Add more water if a thinner drink is desired. Drink immediately. You can use this recipe as a base for experimenting with your favorite seasonal vegetables.

Vegetable Drink No. 2   **Serves 1**

2 carrots, peeled
1 stalk celery
½ cucumber, peeled
2 beet tops
2 cups spring or filtered water

Combine all the ingredients in a blender or food processor and run it on high speed for 60 to 90 seconds or until the drink is totally liquefied. Add more water if a thinner drink is desired. Drink immediately.

Vegetable Drink No. 3   **Serves 1**

2 carrots, peeled
1 stalk celery
½ cup cooked beets
¼ cup parsley
2 cups spring or filtered water

Combine all the ingredients in a blender or food processor and run it on high speed for 60 to 90 seconds or until the drink is totally liquefied. Add more water if a thinner drink is desired. Drink immediately.

Vegetable Juice Cocktail   Serves 4

A healthy twist on a classic. This drink uses purchased organic tomato juice with the freshly juiced vegetables adding additional nutrients. Simply juice the vegetables and add to the tomato juice.

2 cups organic low-sodium tomato or vegetable juice
2 cups spinach
4 carrots
2 stalk of celery
½ green pepper
1 cucumber
¼ cup parsley
½ lemon, peeled

Combine the spinach, cucumber, carrots, celery, lemon, green pepper, parsley and tomato juice in your blender. Garnish with celery stalks and serve right away.

Split-Pea Soup Puree   Serves 2 - 4

1 cup dried split peas, picked over and rinsed
2 carrots
1 onion, chopped
4 cups spring or filtered water
¼ - ½ teaspoon salt or salt substitute

Combine the peas, onion, and carrots in a stockpot. Add water. Bring to a boil, then turn heat to low, and cover pot. Cook for 45 minutes. Add salt and continue cooking until peas are soft. Let soup cool, then puree in a blender or food processor until smooth.

Carrot Soup Puree

Serves 2 - 4

4 cups peeled and sliced carrots
4 cups vegetable broth
2 cups diced onion
½ cup sweet red pepper
1 cup rice or soy milk

Combine all the ingredients in a large stockpot. Cook for 30 minutes a medium heat or until carrots are tender. Let soup cool, then puree in a blender or food processor until smooth.

Butternut Squash Puree

Serves 2 - 4

1 large butternut squash, peeled and cubed
1 teaspoon rice bran syrup
2 cups rice or soy milk
Ground nutmeg, allspice, or cinnamon to taste (optional)

Place the cut squash in a steamer and steam for 12 to 15 minutes or until very tender. While it is still hot, place the steamed squash in a blender or food processor. Add the nondairy milk and rice bran syrup and puree until smooth. Serve hot, with or without spices. This drink tastes like a delicious dessert.

7

The Anti-Fatigue Diet – Step 2: High Nutrient Menus, Meal Plans & Recipes

Once you are starting to feel better, you can greatly expand the range of foods and dishes that you can enjoy. In this chapter I share with you a wide range of delicious menus and recipes that have been created to restore your energy, balance your brain chemistry and hormones and support healthy immunity and digestive function. These meal plans will help you create a foundation of healthful eating during your recovery period and beyond. You can also combine these dishes with foods from Step 1. In fact, if you have mild to moderate fatigue, you may want to mix some of the Step 2 dishes with the Step 1 foods right at the beginning.

Remember that how you feel after eating a meal is the ultimate test of how you are handling foods. You must become your own feedback system to evaluate whether the foods you have selected are helping to relieve your fatigue and elevate your vitality and well-being.

Food has a powerful effect on our energy and mood. I have seen with many of my patients that they were unknowingly eating foods that were contributing to their fatigue and mood related symptoms. For example, many of my patients were eating foods with too much sugar or alcoholic beverages that can worsen chronic fatigue and depression. Sugar and alcohol also worsen moodiness, fatigue and irritability in women who are struggling with PMS and menopause. Some of my patients have had undiagnosed food allergies or intolerances to common foods like milk products and wheat that were worsening their fatigue and tiredness along with other symptoms.

In addition, food fills emotional as well as nutritional needs for many women. For example, women commonly snack on "junk foods" like cookies, colas, candy bars, and other high stress foods when they are feeling stressed out or anxious. While these foods give an immediate emotional boost, the ingredients and additives contained in them often make the fatigue symptoms worse over time.

It is very important to be aware of your specific sensitivities and intolerances to foods when beginning an anti-fatigue program. I have found with my own patients that once they aware of the beneficial role that proper food selection can play in preventing and relieving anxiety and stress, they were always quite motivated to shift their eating habits toward more healthy choices. Most of my patients really enjoyed exploring new, more healthful foods. Best of all, the benefits of choosing foods that boosted their energy and stabilized their mood were often apparent quite quickly, especially when combined with a therapeutic nutritional supplement program.

Making the transition, however, may present some challenges. Many of us tend to be creatures of habit, so the prospect of changing our food selection may sometimes appear difficult and intimidating. Over the years, my patients did best when I provided specific guidelines to help them through the transition period.

When changing from a high stress diet to a chronic fatigue-relief food plan, my patients requested specific menus and meal plans as they began to regain their energy. Although information on which foods to eat and which to avoid is tremendously helpful, most women want to know how to take the next step and combine the right foods in healthful meals. Many of my patients benefited enormously from these simple and easy-to-follow guidelines, so I have included the information in this chapter for your benefit, too

Unfortunately, most cookbooks do not adequately address a woman's needs for specific nutrients when they are suffering from chronic fatigue and depression. Many contain recipes that are too high in the nutrients that can worsen mood imbalances such as sugar, caffeine, alcohol, chocolate, animal fats, dairy products and too much salt.

Many nutrition-conscious cookbooks present low-calorie "light dishes" that eliminate the high stress ingredients, but still don't give women suffering from fatigue and depression the therapeutic levels of specific nutrients they need. To help with this issue, I have also created a number of recipes that I have included in this chapter to further support your transition towards restoring your energy and vitality. My patients have found this extremely beneficial and have given me very positive feedback about their enjoyment of many of these dishes as well as receiving beneficial therapeutic results. My own friends and family have also greatly enjoyed these healthy dishes and meals over the years.

I have found that no one diet fits the needs of all different body types. Because of this I have included menus and delicious recipes for women who prefer a vegetarian emphasis, high complex carbohydrate diet as well as dishes and entrees for women who feel their best on a high protein meat-based diet. All of these meal plans and recipes contain ingredients most suitable for providing relief for women with fatigue and depression. In addition, the high stress ingredients that can worsen your symptoms have been eliminated.

Because too elaborate food preparation can be difficult for women who are struggling with fatigue, I've devised recipes that are quick and easy to prepare. I have found that anything too complicated doesn't work for many of my patients. Best of all, these recipes are delicious as well as healthful. I hope that you find trying these new dishes to be a delightful adventure as well.

As previously mentioned, I have found that no one diet fits the needs of all different body types. Because of this I have included menus and delicious recipes for women who prefer a vegetarian emphasis, high complex carbohydrate diet as well as dishes and entrees for women who feel their best on a high protein, meat-based diet. All of these meal plans and recipes contain ingredients most suitable for providing relief for women suffering from chronic fatigue, tiredness and depression. In addition, the high stress ingredients that can worsen your symptoms have been eliminated.

Breakfast Menus

These breakfast menus have been developed to help reduce symptoms of fatigue and depression during the recovery phase. All the dishes contain high levels of the essential nutrients that women with these problems need. The recipes call for no high stress ingredients. Healthful and nourishing foods will provide the energy and vitality you need to sail through your work and activities. You can use these as idea generators for your own meal planning.

Breakfast has been one of the easiest meals for my patients to restructure along healthier lines. It tends to be a smaller and simpler meal. You may want to make healthful dietary changes in your breakfast first and then move on to lunch and dinner.

Flax shake with protein powder and fresh fruit

~~~~~~~~~~~~~

Blueberry and green food smoothie

~~~~~~~~~~~~~

Millet cereal with raisins and cinnamon
Nondairy yogurt
Chamomile tea

~~~~~~~~~~~~~

Rice and flaxseed pancakes
Banana
Vanilla nondairy milk

~~~~~~~~~~~~~

Oatmeal with raspberries
Chamomile tea

~~~~~~~~~~~~~

Nondairy yogurt with granola and ground flaxseed
Peppermint tea

~~~~~~~~~~~~~

Omelette with chicken sausage
Roasted grain beverage (coffee substitute)

~~~~~~~~~~~~~

Scrambled eggs and turkey bacon
Ginger tea

~~~~~~~~~~~~~

Lunch and Dinner Menus

I have included a variety of menus you can choose from when planning your meals. You can use these menu plans for meals, or as idea generators to fit your own taste and needs. These dishes contain many nutritious and healthful ingredients for relief of fatigue and depression.

Use these menus as helpful guidelines throughout the entire month. Your nutritional status on a day-by-day basis determines in part how likely you are to have fatigue symptoms. These dishes should help to diminish the severity of your symptoms because they eliminate high stress foods.

Soup Meals
Split pea soup
Pumpkin muffins
Fresh applesauce
~~~~~~~~~~~~~~~

Chicken and wild rice soup
Cole slaw
Millet bread with flaxseed oil
~~~~~~~~~~~~~~~

Vegetable soup with brown rice
Steamed kale
Baked potato with flaxseed oil
Apple slices
~~~~~~~~~~~~~~~

Lentil soup
Herbed brown rice
Broccoli with lemon
~~~~~~~~~~~~~~~

Tomato soup
Potato salad with low-fat mayonnaise
Celery and carrot sticks
~~~~~~~~~~~~~~~

Salad Meals
Spinach salad with turkey bacon or tofu
Corn muffins with flaxseed oil
Orange slices
~~~~~~~~~~~~~~~

Beet salad with goat cheese
Rice crackers with fresh fruit preserves
~~~~~~~~~~~~~~~

Romaine salad with grilled salmon
Gluten-free bread and olive oil dip
~~~~~~~~~~~~~~~

Low-fat potato salad
Cole slaw
Hard boiled eggs
Melon slices
~~~~~~~~~~~~~~~

Mixed Vegetable Salad with Garbanzo Beans
Baked yam with flaxseed oil and cinnamon

Meat Meals

Poached salmon with lemon
Herbed brown rice
Steamed carrots with honey

~~~~~~~~~~~~~~

Roasted chicken with herbs
Baked potato with flaxseed oil
Broccoli with lemon

~~~~~~~~~~~~~~

Broiled trout with dill
Mixed green salad with vinaigrette
Green peas and onions
Apple slices

~~~~~~~~~~~~~~

Grilled shrimp with olive oil and lemon
Wild rice
Steamed kale

~~~~~~~~~~~~~~

One-Dish Vegetable Meals

Vegetarian tacos with black beans, brown rice, avocados and low-salt salsa

~~~~~~~~~~~~~~

Stir-fry with mixed vegetables, brown rice and tofu
Orange slices

~~~~~~~~~~~~~~

Pasta with tomato sauce, broccoli, carrots, olive oil and garlic
Green salad with vinaigrette

~~~~~~~~~~~~~~

Hummus dip
Eggplant dip (babaganoush)
Mixed raw vegetable slices including carrots, red bell peppers, and radishes

~~~~~~~~~~~~~~

Brown rice and almond tabouli
Mixed olives
Melon slices

~~~~~~~~~~~~~~

Breakfast Recipes

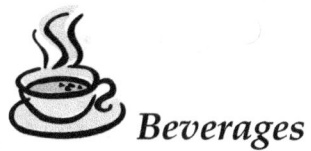 *Beverages*

These drinks are made with therapeutic herbal teas, power smoothies that are rich in fruits, raw seeds, nuts, protein powder, green foods and nondairy milk that are recommended for preventing and treating your symptoms. The ingredients contain high levels of essential nutrients that help support healthy brain chemistry and hormonal balance and relax tension in the muscles.

Feel Good Herb Tea   **Serves 2**

2 cups water
1 teaspoon chamomile leaves
1 teaspoon peppermint leaves
½ teaspoon honey (if desired)

Bring the water to a boil. Place herbs in water and stir. Turn heat to low and simmer for 15 minutes.

Peppermint and chamomile are both muscle relaxants and antispasmodic herbs, so they can provide relief of pain and cramping. They help balance the mood and provide deep restful sleep if your fatigue is due, in part, to insomnia.

Ginger Tea **Serves 4**

Ginger makes a warming, delicious tea and is beneficial to your circulation. It is also a powerful anti-inflammatory herb. If the tea is too strong add more water.

5 cups water
3 tablespoons ginger coarsely chopped
½ lemon (optional)
Honey (or other sweetener, to taste)

Add ginger to the water in a cooking pot. Bring to a boil and then turn heat to low. Steep for 15 or 20 minutes. Squeeze lemon into tea and serve with honey or your favorite sweetener.

Vitality Herb Tea **Serves 2**

2 cups water
1 teaspoon green tea leaves
1 teaspoon peppermint leaves
½ teaspoon honey (if desired)

Bring the water to a boil. Place herbs in water and stir. Turn heat to low and simmer for 15 minutes.

This is a very beneficial combination for the relief of fatigue and tiredness. Green tea contains a very small amount of caffeine along with many other health benefits.

Simple Flax Smoothie   Serves 2

Flaxseed is not only a tasty addition to smoothies but it is also very nutritious. Flaxseed is high in essential fatty acids, calcium, magnesium, and potassium.

1 cup vanilla nondairy milk
2 tablespoons ground flaxseed
1 banana

Combine all ingredients in a blender. Blend until smooth and serve.

Raspberry Flax Smoothie   Serves 2

This creamy smoothie makes a great breakfast. Flaxseed oil one is my favorite foods. It is both delicious and rich in healthy omega-3 fatty acids. It also adds extra creaminess to the smoothie.

1 cup rice milk
¾ cup raspberries – fresh or frozen
1 heaping tablespoon rice protein powder
1 tablespoon flaxseed oil
2 bananas, sliced

Combine all ingredients in a blender. Puree until smooth and serve.

Heavenly Strawberry Coconut Smoothie   Serves 2

This drink fits its name! It is absolutely scrumptious as well as good for you. If you don't have a high-speed blender and you are using whole raw cashews I recommend that you chop them up beforehand. Otherwise raw cashew butter is a good substitute.

1 cup Coconut Dream, unsweetened
1 cup strawberries – fresh or frozen
1 tablespoon raw coconut flour
2 tablespoons raw cashews (10-15)
1 banana, sliced

Combine all ingredients in a blender. Puree until smooth and serve.

Blueberry Coconut Smoothie **Serves 2**

1 cup coconut water
¾ cup blueberries – fresh or frozen
1 heaping tablespoon raw coconut flour
1 heaping tablespoon raw almonds (10-15)
1 banana, sliced

Combine all ingredients in a blender. Puree until smooth and serve.

Delicious Green Drink **Serves 1**

½ cup Concord grape juice
¼ cup water
1 tablespoon ground flaxseed
½ teaspoon chlorella powder
½ teaspoon spirulina powder

Mix all ingredients together in a glass or puree in a blender.

Blueberry and Greens Shake **Serves 2**

This drink is a powerhouse of nutrients! The chlorella and spirulina are highly beneficial green foods. They are rich in nutrients like beta-carotene and help to detoxify the liver. They are readily available at health food stores.

1 cup nondairy milk
¾ cup blueberries – fresh or frozen
2 tablespoons protein powder
½ teaspoon chlorella
½ teaspoon spirulina
Sprinkle of Truvia (optional)

In a blender puree the nondairy milk and blueberries. Add the rest of ingredients and blend well.

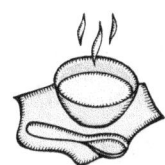 *Healthy, Quick Breakfasts*

Most American breakfasts include wheat and dairy products, such as yogurt, wheat toast, wheat cereal with milk, sweet rolls, and other wheat-based pastries. As I explained earlier in this book, dairy products and wheat can worsen the symptoms of fatigue and depression. Gluten and casein, the proteins found in wheat and milk, can trigger symptoms of mood imbalances, bloating, digestive disturbances and fatigue.

I have included in this section both whole grain, carbohydrate-based entrees as well as protein-rich dishes, depending on the type of diet that makes you feel your best. Both types of entrees, however, will benefit fatigue symptoms by eliminating wheat and dairy products at breakfast.

The whole grain dishes are based on ground flaxseed, gluten-free grains and soy (if tolerated), all of which can be useful in reducing your symptoms. The protein-rich entrees have been created using eggs and healthy breakfast meats. The smoothies also contain protein powder.

Quinoa Cereal with Strawberries   **Serves 2**

1 ½ cups cooked quinoa
1 cup nondairy milk
½ cup strawberries
2 teaspoons honey or other sweetener

Combine quinoa and nondairy milk in a saucepan. Simmer for 5 minutes. Stir in honey and garnish with raspberries.

Quinoa with Prunes   Serves 2

This is one of my all-time favorite hot cereals. The plums are delicious and add a nice texture. Quinoa is a small, protein rich grain. When cooked the grains are small and fluffy. I recommend making a pot of quinoa the night before.

1 ½ cups cooked quinoa
1 cup nondairy milk
4-6 dried prunes, chopped
2 tablespoons flaxseed oil
2 teaspoons xylitol, honey, or maple syrup (if using unsweetened milk)
Pinch of salt (optional)

In a saucepan combine quinoa, nondairy milk, salt, and dried plums. Heat thoroughly and simmer on low heat for 5-10 minutes until plums have softened. Serve with flaxseed oil and sweetener.

Maple Cinnamon Oatmeal   Serves 2

1 cup gluten-free quick oats
1 ¾ cups water
1-2 tablespoons flaxseed oil
2 teaspoons maple syrup
Pinch of cinnamon (to taste)
Pinch of salt

Boil water in a saucepan. Add gluten-free oats and reduce to medium heat. Cook for one minute and stir. Cover, and remove oatmeal from heat. Serve in 2-3 minutes. Stir in maple syrup, flaxseed oil, cinnamon and salt.

Strawberries and Cream Oatmeal   Serves 2

1 cup gluten-free quick oats
½ cup strawberries, chopped
½ nondairy milk
1 ¼ cups water
1-2 tablespoons flaxseed oil
2 teaspoons honey or stevia
Pinch of salt (optional)

Bring water and nondairy milk to a boil in a saucepan. Add gluten-free oats and reduce to medium heat. Cook for one minute and stir. Cover, and remove oatmeal from heat. Serve in 2-3 minutes. Stir in sweetener, flaxseed oil, salt and top with strawberries.

Banana Nut Muffins   Makes 14-18

These moist muffins are a twist on the classic recipe using cashews instead of walnuts. Very tasty!

1½ cups rice flour
1 teaspoon baking powder
½ teaspoon baking soda
3 ripe bananas, mashed
¼ teaspoon cinnamon
6 packets of Truvia (¼ cup)
¼ cup honey
¼ cup safflower oil
¼ cup cashews, chopped

Preheat oven to 350 degrees. Mix all dry ingredients and wet ingredients separately. Combine and mix well. Fill muffin cups ¾ with batter.

Pumpkin Muffins

Makes 14-18 muffins

1½ cups rice flour
½ teaspoon baking powder
½ teaspoon baking soda
1 cup pumpkin
1 teaspoon cinnamon
¼ teaspoon nutmeg
¼ cup chopped almonds (optional)
3 tablespoons molasses
3 tablespoons safflower oil
½ cup raisins
2 eggs
½ cup nondairy milk
1 teaspoon vanilla extract
Pinch of salt

Preheat oven to 400 degrees. Line a muffin tin with paper muffin cups.

Combine all dry ingredients and mix thoroughly. In a separate bowl beat the two eggs and then combine the remainder of the wet ingredients. Add the wet ingredients to the dry and mix thoroughly.

Fill muffin cups ¾ with batter. Cook for 18-20 minutes or until thoroughly cooked.

Flaxseed Pancakes   **Makes 8 pancakes (serves 2-4)**

Xylitol is an excellent sugar substitute for cooking and baking that can be found at most health food stores. Xylitol is easy to use because it has a 1:1 ratio with sugar. Yet, this product has 40% fewer calories than sugar and is beneficial for your teeth and gums.

1 cup gluten-free flour
1 cup unsweetened rice milk
1 egg
2 tablespoons xylitol
1 tablespoon ground flaxseed
1 teaspoon baking powder
½ teaspoon baking soda
¼ teaspoon salt
3 tablespoons almond oil, keeping 1 tbsp. for cooking
Maple syrup (optional)
Fruit jam (optional)

Mix the dry and wet ingredients in separate bowls. Combine all the ingredients and mix thoroughly. Cook on medium heat and use a small amount of oil to grease the pan if needed. When pancakes bubble in the center flip and cook for 1-2 minutes until cooked thoroughly. Serve with maple syrup or all-fruit jam. Delicious!

Egg and Sausage Scramble **Serves 2**

4 eggs
4 turkey breakfast sausages
2 slice of gluten-free toast
Salt and pepper (optional)
2 teaspoons olive oil
Serve with ½ cup applesauce

Warm a frying pan on medium heat and add olive oil. Beat egg gently in a small bowl and set aside. Chop the sausages into small pieces - this will help them to cook faster. Add sausages to the pan and cook for several minutes until sausages are brown.

Turn heat to low and add eggs to the pan and scramble with the sausage. Add a pinch of salt and pepper. Serve with toast and applesauce. Bake for 20-25 minutes until cooked through.

Mushroom Onion Scramble **Serves 2**

The mushrooms and onion give this egg scramble a great texture. The water helps make the eggs fluffier.

4 eggs
1 tablespoon water
¼ onion
2-3 mushrooms
1 tablespoon olive oil
Salt and pepper (optional)

Dice the mushrooms and onion. Next, beat the 4 eggs together with 1 tablespoon water. Preheat the frying pan on medium heat and add 1 tablespoon olive oil. Add onion and mushroom and cook for about 3 minutes until onions are translucent and add eggs. Let sit for about 30 second and then start to scramble with your spatula. Add a pinch of salt and pepper and serve.

Spinach and Tomato Scramble   **Serves 2**

The sprinkle of Parmesan cheese adds a delightful saltiness and tang to this dish.

4 eggs, beaten
1 tablespoon water
2 tablespoons diced onion
¼ tomato, chopped
12 spinach leaves, chopped
1 tablespoon olive oil
Salt and pepper (optional)
Parmesan cheese - or soy Parmesan (optional)

Beat the 4 eggs together with 1 tablespoon water. Preheat the frying pan on medium heat and add 1 tablespoon olive oil. Add onion and cook for about 3 minutes until onions are translucent. Next add eggs, spinach and tomato. Let sit for about 15 seconds and then start to scramble with your spatula. Sprinkle on a small amount of Parmesan cheese, add a pinch of salt and pepper and serve.

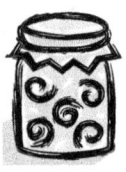 *Spreads and Sauces*

These spreads and sauces contain highly concentrated levels of ingredients that help to improve energy and balance blood sugar levels. Serve with rice cakes, crackers, corn bread, or even spread on a banana for a delicious treat.

Fresh Applesauce   Serves 2

2 ½ apples
½ cup fresh apple juice
½ teaspoon cinnamon
½ teaspoon ginger

Peel apples and cut into quarters; remove cores. Combine all ingredients in a food processor. Blend until smooth.

Sesame-Tofu Spread   Serves 4

¼ cup soft tofu
¼ cup raw sesame butter
¼ cup honey

Combine all ingredients in a blender. Serve with rice cakes or crackers.

Lunch and Dinner Recipes

These high-nutrient, healthful lunch and dinner dishes are designed to help relieve fatigue and balance your mood. The ingredients do not include red meat, dairy products, or wheat, all of which can worsen your symptoms. Mix and match these dishes as you please. You might combine soups and salads or whole grains, legumes and vegetables for a complete vegetarian emphasis or meat-based meal, depending on your needs for carbohydrates and protein.

The main course dishes are all extremely healthful for women with chronic fatigue. They are rich in essential nutrients that will help to boost your energy and vitality.

 *Soups*

Split Pea Soup   **Serves 4**

¾ cup split peas
5 cups low-sodium chicken broth
¾ cup carrot, chopped
¾ cup onion, diced
Tamari soy sauce – to taste (optional)

Bring the water to a boil and add the split peas, onion, carrots, and chicken broth. Reduce heat to low and simmer for 50 minutes – 1 hour, stirring occasionally. If water begins to cook off add up to an extra cup of water. Add a dash of tamari soy sauce for a saltier flavor.

Black Bean Soup   **Serves 4**

This recipe is easy and makes a delicious, filling soup.

1 can black beans (14 ounce), rinsed
5 cups low-sodium vegetable broth
1 cup onion, diced
¾ cup carrot, chopped
¾ cup red pepper, chopped
¼ teaspoon cumin
Tamari soy sauce – to taste (optional)

Bring the water to a boil and add all ingredients. Reduce heat to low and simmer for 30 minutes, stirring occasionally. If water begins to cook off add up to an extra cup of water. Add a dash of tamari soy sauce for a saltier flavor.

Chicken Rice Soup   **Serves 4-6**

Few things make me feel better than a bowl of homemade chicken rice soup. I have an easy tip to add extra flavor to your soup: If you used the meat from a roasted, skin-on chicken you can add some of the skin to the soup while it is cooking. This will add depth and richness to your soup. Remove the skin when the soup has finished cooking.

6 cups low-sodium chicken broth
¾ cup carrot
1 cup celery, diced
1 cup cooked chicken, diced
¾ cup onion, diced
¾ cup brown rice, cooked
Tamari soy sauce – to taste (optional)

Bring water to a boil and add all ingredients. Reduce heat to low and simmer for 30 minutes, stirring occasionally. If water begins to cook off add up to an extra cup of water. Add a dash of tamari soy sauce for a saltier flavor.

Butternut Squash Soup   **Serves 4**

This soup has been a long-time favorite of mine. I adore the light, creamy texture. Adding maple syrup enhances the natural sweetness of the squash.

½ onion, diced
1 cup low-sodium chicken broth
2 cups pureed butternut squash - fresh or frozen (fresh is preferred)
½ teaspoon cinnamon
1½ cups nondairy milk
2 teaspoons maple syrup
1 tablespoon safflower oil
½-¾ teaspoon salt

In a large saucepan heat the oil on medium heat. Add the onion and cook until translucent. Add the butternut squash, chicken broth, cinnamon and salt. Mix well and simmer for 5 minutes. Add nondairy milk and maple syrup. Simmer on low heat for ten minutes. Stir frequently while cooking the soup.

Optional: To make extra creamy, blend the soup when it has finished cooking. Wait for the soup to cool before blending.

 *Salads*

Zingy Watercress Salad Serves 4

I enjoy the refreshing bitterness of watercress. This salad pairs well with green apple. Watercress has a strong flavor and a little goes a long way.

1 cup watercress, coarsely chopped
4 cups butter lettuce (or other soft lettuce), coarsely chopped
2 teaspoons scallions, finely chopped
½ green apple, chopped
1 ounce goat cheese, crumbled
Vinaigrette dressing

In a large bowl toss the watercress, butter lettuce, green onion, and apple together with the vinaigrette dressing (to taste). On top of the salad crumble the goat cheese.

Scrumptious Veggie Salad Serves 4-6

This is one of my favorite salads! It pairs wonderfully with soups and sandwiches.

1 head red lettuce, chopped into bite size pieces
1 large tomato, chopped
2 green onions, sliced
6 mushrooms, sliced
¾ cup kidney beans – canned works well
1 avocado, sliced
¼ cup sunflower seeds
Vinaigrette dressing (to taste)

Combine all ingredients except for avocado in a large salad bowl. Mix in Vinaigrette dressing and top with avocado slices before serving.

Potato Salad **Serves 4-6**

This is a light twist on classic potato salad and makes a great side dish. The vegetables add a delightful crunchiness. This salad pairs well with a turkey or chicken sandwich.

10-12 small red potatoes, cut into bite size pieces (about 2 cups)
2 tablespoons diced celery
2 tablespoons diced red onion
2 tablespoons diced red pepper
1 heaping tablespoon diced water chestnuts
1 hardboiled egg, yolk removed
1 heaping tablespoon mayonnaise
1 teaspoon whole grain Dijon mustard

Steam the potatoes for 15-20 minutes or until fork tender and let cool. Chop up all the vegetables into small pieces and set aside. Chop egg white and set aside. In a mixing bowl add vegetables, mayonnaise and mustard to the potatoes and mix well. Add egg, mix, and serve.

Radicchio and Orange Salad **Serves 4-6**

This is a sophisticated and delicious salad. I love salads with "extras" such as fruit or a little bit of goat cheese.

6 cups salad greens
½ radicchio, sliced thin
¼ red onion, sliced very thin
3 ounces goat cheese
1 medium sized orange, peeled and cut into bite size segments
Orange vinaigrette

In a large bowl combine salad greens, radicchio, onion, and oranges. Pour vinaigrette, to taste, over salad and toss. Add goat cheese before serving.

Caesar Salad **Serves 2-4**

I love Caesar salads. They have been my favorite salad for years! The crispy romaine lettuce and creamy Caesar dressing is a perfect match. I like to use anchovies because they are delicious in this salad and also full of healthy anti-inflammatory oils. I prefer the filets packed in olive oil.

1 head of romaine lettuce, chopped – about 6 cups
4 tablespoons light Caesar dressing
4 anchovy filets, chopped
¾ cup gluten-free croutons
1½ teaspoons grated Parmesan cheese
1 cup roast chicken, cubed (optional)

In a large mixing bowl pour your favorite Caesar's dressing over lettuce. Mix well so that leaves are evenly coated with dressing. Add croutons, Parmesan cheese, anchovies, and toss well. Top with roasted chicken and serve.

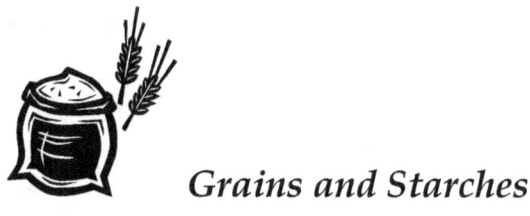

Grains and Starches

Wild Rice   **Serves 2**

¾ cup wild rice
2 ½ cups water
½ teaspoon salt

Wash rice with cold water. Combine all ingredients in a cooking pot and bring to a rapid boil. Turn flame to low, cover, and cook without stirring (about 45 minutes) until rice is tender but not mushy. Uncover and fluff with a fork. Cook an additional 5 minutes, and then serve.

Kasha   **Serves 4**

1 cup kasha (buckwheat groats)
3 ¼ cups water
Pinch of salt

Bring ingredients to a boil, lower heat, and simmer for 25 minutes or until soft. The grains should be fluffy, like rice. *For breakfast, blend in blender with water until creamy. Add almond milk, sesame milk, or sunflower milk, and cinnamon, apple butter, raisins, or berries.*

Delicious Baked Sweet Potato   Serves 4

4 sweet potatoes
1 teaspoon olive oil
1 tablespoon flax oil for each potato

Preheat oven to 400° F. Wash the potatoes, then rub with olive oil. Bake for 45 to 60 minutes, or until soft when pierced with a fork. Garnish with flax oil. Honey, maple syrup, or chopped raw pecans may also be used.

Baked Potato   Serves 4

4 russet or Idaho potatoes
2 teaspoons olive oil
1 tablespoon flax oil for each potato

Preheat oven to 400° F. Wash the potatoes, rub them with olive oil, and bake for 45 to 60 minutes, or until soft when pierced with a fork. Garnish with flax oil. Other garnishes can include chopped green onions, soy cheese, and salsa.

Vegetables

Kale with Lemon   Serves 4

Kale is one of my favorite vegetables and it also has terrific health benefits for women since it is a good source of calcium and other essential nutrients like lutein that supports your hormonal health and the health of your heart and eyes.

1 bunch of kale
1 lemon, cut into quarters
Soy sauce

Rinse kale well and remove stems. Steam for 5-6 minutes or until leaves wilt and are tender. Dress lightly with soy sauce and lemon juice.

Jessica's Favorite Broccoli   Serves 4

1 pound broccoli
1 tablespoons flaxseed oil
Pinch of salt (optional)
Squeeze of lemon

Cut the broccoli into small florets; steam until tender. Squeeze lemon juice over broccoli and add the flax oil. Mix and serve.

Cauliflower with Flaxseed Oil   Serves 4

1 medium head cauliflower
2 tablespoons flaxseed oil
Pinch of salt (optional)

Break the cauliflower into small florets. Steam until tender. Toss with flax oil and salt.

Cranberry Almond Brussels Sprouts   Serves 2-4

The dried cranberries in this dish really make it special by adding a touch of tangy sweetness. Cranberries are high in energy enhancing vitamin C.

2 cups Brussels sprouts, chopped into bite size pieces
2 tablespoons slivered almonds
2 tablespoons dried cranberries, coarsely chopped
1 teaspoon almond oil
Pinch of salt

Steam Brussels sprouts for 5-7 minutes, until slightly tender but retaining their color.

In a frying pan, heat the oil on medium-low. Add almonds and stir until they begin to turn light brown. Add cranberries and continue cooking for 15-30 seconds. Take the pan off the heat and add Brussels sprouts.

Combine the Brussels sprouts, almonds and cranberries, cook for a minute and serve.

Honey Carrots   Serves 4

This is one of my favorite side dishes. The warm honey brings out the natural sweetness of the carrots.

3 cups carrots, sliced thin
1 teaspoon honey
1 teaspoon almond oil
Pinch of salt (optional)

Cut carrots into thin slices and steam for 6-8 minutes, or until tender. Using the same saucepan pour out the cooking water and on low heat add the honey and oil and mix well. Add carrots and mix all ingredients together. Add a pinch of salt before serving.

Roasted Rosemary Potatoes   **Serves 4-6**

I love roasted potatoes! This is a wonderful potato recipe that I like to make when I serve roasted chicken.

4 cups red potatoes – about 4 or 5 large red potatoes
1 tablespoon dried rosemary, crushed
3 tablespoons of olive oil
2 garlic cloves, minced
¼ teaspoon black pepper (optional)
Pinch of salt

Preheat oven to 400 degrees. Cut potatoes into bite size pieces and put into plastic bag. Add olive oil, rosemary, garlic, and black pepper to bag. Close bag and shake to coat all of the potato pieces. Line a baking tray with foil and put potatoes on to tray. Arrange evenly in one layer.

Sprinkle salt onto potatoes and bake for 30-35 minutes until brown and cooked through. During cooking stir the potatoes once if desired.

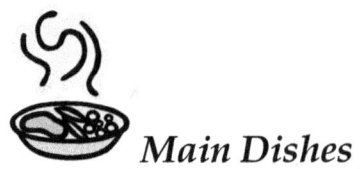 *Main Dishes*

Mega Greens Rice Bowl   **Serves 4**

This dish is a satisfying way to get a large serving of healthy greens. A delicious sauce is Organicville's Island Teriyaki (organicvillefoods.com). Their sauce is made with agave nectar instead of cane sugar.

4 cups kale, cut into bite size pieces (about ½ bunch)
3 cups baby bok choy, chopped
1 cup of white mushrooms, sliced
1 carrot, finely chopped
8 ounces of tofu, cubed
3 cups cooked brown rice - ¾ cup rice per person
Teriyaki sauce – soy sauce - gomasio

Steam the carrots for 4 minutes and then add the kale, bok choy, mushrooms, and tofu. Steam for 5 minutes. Serve in a deep bowl over rice with your choice of sauce.

Good sauces for this dish include teriyaki sauce and soy sauce. A little bit of lemon juice and gomasio also works well.

Baked Tofu Rice Bowl **Serves 4**

Baked tofu has a rich, nutty flavor that I love. This recipe is fun but also very tasty and rich in healthy greens. I always make sure that the vegetables are cut into bite size pieces.

3 cups broccoli, chopped
3 cups baby bok choy, chopped
1 carrot, finely chopped
½ cup mushrooms, sliced
½ cup red pepper
Baked tofu
3 cups cooked brown rice - ¾ cup rice per person

Steam the carrots for 4 minutes and then add the broccoli, baby bok choy, mushrooms, and red pepper. Steam for 5 minutes. Serve in a deep bowl over rice with your choice of sauce. Layer a few pieces of baked tofu on top.

Summertime Veggie Pasta   **Serves 4**

This light pasta is one of my favorite dishes to eat during the summer. The pasta and sauce are light but filling. It's a dish that I love to share to share with friends.

1 box quinoa elbow pasta (8 ounce box)
½ onion, diced
2 cans Italian seasoned diced tomatoes
1 can garbanzo beans
1 carrot, shredded
1½ cups cooked Brussels sprouts or broccoli
½ teaspoon dried basil
2 teaspoons olive oil
Pinch of pepper
Pinch of salt (optional)

Cook pasta according to package directions. In a saucepan on medium heat add olive oil and onions. Sautee until onions are translucent. Add remainder of ingredients and bring to a simmer. Cook on low heat for 10 minutes. Combine the cooked noodles with the sauce.

Mushroom and Eggplant Sandwich   **Serves 2**

This sandwich is a variation on the open-face mushroom sandwich. This sandwich uses eggplant spread instead of mayonnaise and mustard, which gives the sandwich a delightful spiciness. I like the Eggplant Garlic Spread from Trader Joe's. This sandwich is also best served open-face.

4 slices gluten-free bread
4 cups mushrooms, sliced – *I prefer basic white mushrooms*
1½ cups mixed greens
½ tomato, sliced thin
1 teaspoon balsamic vinegar
1 tablespoon olive oil
2 tablespoons eggplant spread
Pinch of salt
Pinch of pepper

Warm a frying pan on medium heat and add olive oil. Add mushrooms and sauté gently adding a generous pinch of salt and pepper. When mushrooms begin to cook down turn heat to low and add balsamic vinegar. Continue to cook until mushrooms are soft and begin to lightly brown. Total cooking time is about 6-8 minutes.

Toast bread and spread on the eggplant spread. Dress each piece of bread with the greens and a slice or two of tomato. Spoon the cooked mushrooms on to each slice of bread.

Parmesan Chicken Pasta   **Serves 4**

This dish is a crowd pleaser that I often serve when I have friends over. The sprinkle of Parmesan cheese adds a delightful tanginess that rounds out the dish perfectly.

6 cups gluten-free pasta, cooked
1 ½ cups roasted chicken, cubed
¾ cup diced carrots
¾ cup diced red onion
½ onion, diced
1 small tomato, finely chopped
3 cups broccoli, chopped into bite size pieces
¾ cup chicken broth (recommended) or water
1 teaspoon dried basil
1 tablespoon olive oil
Soy Parmesan cheese or regular, grated
Generous pinch of pepper
Pinch of salt (optional)

In a frying pan on medium heat add the olive oil. Add the onion and sauté until onion begin to turn translucent. Add all vegetables except tomatoes and cook for 1-2 minutes. Add chicken broth, chicken, tomatoes, basil, and pepper. Turn heat to low, cover and simmer for 5-7 minutes or until broth has cooked down. Add more broth if needed.

Add the sauce to the pasta. Serve with Parmesan cheese.

Turkey Bolognese **Serves 2-4**

This dish cooks up quickly and is very satisfying. This is a versatile recipe. You can add all kinds of vegetables and it will taste great.

½ lb. ground turkey
2 cans of diced tomatoes
1 can tomato paste
½ onion, diced
1 carrot, diced
1 zucchini, diced
1 teaspoon basil
1 teaspoon oregano
1 tablespoon olive oil
¼ teaspoon salt (optional)
½ teaspoon black pepper (optional)
Water (optional)

Heat pan on medium and add olive oil. Add onion and sauté until translucent. Add turkey and all herbs and spices. Cook until turkey has browned and cooked thoroughly. Add tomatoes, tomato paste, carrots, and zucchini. Cook on low heat for 12-15 minutes. If sauce is too thick add a small amount of water until desired consistency is reached. Serve over brown rice spaghetti.

Simple Broiled Tuna   Serves 4

4 fillets of tuna, 4 ounces each
2 teaspoons olive oil
Squeeze of lemon juice
Pinch of salt

Baste the tuna fillets with oil; then sprinkle with lemon juice. Place tuna in a broiler pan and broil until the level of doneness that you prefer (rare or well-done).

Simple Steamed Salmon   Serves 4

4 fillets of salmon, 4 ounces each
1 cup water
Squeeze of lemon

Combine water and lemon juice in a steamer. Place salmon fillets in streamer basket. Cook to the level of doneness that you prefer.

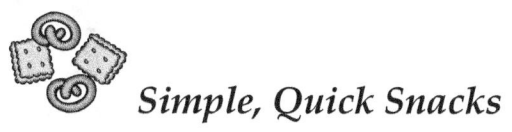 *Simple, Quick Snacks*

Trail Mix **Makes ¾ cup**

¼ cup raw unsalted pumpkin seeds

¼ cup raw unsalted sunflower seeds

¼ cup raisins

Combine and store in a container in the refrigerator. This trail mix is very high in essential fatty acids, calcium, magnesium, and iron. I use it for a snack food to replace stressful and unhealthy sugar-based sweets and chocolate. It is a great mix to take on trips, and I eat it often for breakfast.

Rice Cakes with Nut Butter and Jam **Serves 2**

4 unsalted rice cakes

2 tablespoons raw almond butter

2 tablespoons fruit preserves (no sugar added)

Spread rice cakes with almond butter and fruit preserves for a quick snack.

Herbal tea makes a good accompaniment.

Rice Cakes with Tuna Fish **Serves 2**

4 unsalted rice cakes

4 ounces tuna fish

1 teaspoon low-calorie mayonnaise

Spread rice cakes with tuna fish and mayonnaise.

This is an excellent high-protein snack.

Apple with Almond Butter   Serves 2

1 apple, sliced
1 tablespoon raw almond butter

Spread almond butter on thin apple slices.

Banana with Sesame Butter   Serves 2

1 banana, halved
1 tablespoon raw sesame butter

Spread sesame butter on each half of a ripe banana.

Substitute Healthy Ingredients in Recipes

Learning how to make substitutions for high-stress ingredients in familiar recipes allows you to make your favorite foods without compromising your energy level and vitality. Many recipes contain ingredients that women with chronic fatigue must avoid - dairy products, alcohol, sugar, chocolate, and wheat flour. By eliminating the high stress foods and replacing them with healthier ingredients, you can continue to make many recipes that appeal to you. I have recommended this approach for years to my patients, who are pleased to find that they can still have their favorite dishes, but in much healthier versions.

Some women choose to totally eliminate high stress ingredients from a recipe. For example, you can make a pasta dish with tomato sauce, but eliminate the Parmesan cheese topping and use gluten-free pasta. Greek salad can be made without the feta cheese. Some of my patients even make pizza without cheese, layering tomato sauce and lots of vegetables on the crust. In many cases, the high stress ingredients are not necessary to make foods taste good. Always remember that they can worsen your fatigue symptoms.

If you want to retain a particular high stress ingredient, you can usually substantially reduce the amount of that ingredient you use, while still retaining the flavor and taste. Most of us have palates jaded by too much fat, salt, sugar, and other flavorings. In many dishes, we taste only the additives; we never really enjoy the delicious flavors of the foods themselves.

Now that I regularly substitute low-stress ingredients in my cooking, I find that I enjoy the subtle taste of the dishes much more. Also, I find that my health and vitality continue to improve with the removal of high stress ingredients from my diet. The following information tells you how to substitute healthy ingredients in your own recipes. The substitutions are simple to make and should benefit your health greatly.

How to Substitute for Caffeinated Foods and Beverages

Drink substitutes for coffee and black tea. The best substitutes are the grain-based coffee beverages, such as Postum and Cafix. Some women may find the abrupt discontinuance of coffee too difficult because of withdrawal symptoms, such as headaches. If this concerns you, decrease your total coffee intake gradually to only one or one-half cup per day. Use coffee substitutes for your other cups. This will help prevent withdrawal symptoms.

Use decaffeinated coffee or tea as a transition beverage. If you cannot give up coffee, start by substituting water processed decaffeinated coffee for the real thing. Then try to wean yourself from coffee altogether, or go to a coffee substitute.

Use herbal teas for energy and vitality. Many women with chronic fatigue mistakenly drink coffee as a pick-me-up to be able to function during the day. Use peppermint or ginger teas instead. These teas are energizing but won't have a negative effect on your mood. If you can handle a small amount of caffeine, then green tea is a great option. It has a slight stimulant effect as well as many other health benefits. To make ginger tea, grate a few teaspoons of fresh ginger root into a pot of hot water; boil and steep.

Substitute carob for chocolate. Chocolate can be an issue if you are suffering from fatigue and tiredness because it contains both small amounts of caffeine and quite a bit of sugar for flavoring since cocoa is inherently bitter tasting. If you have a chocolate habit and find that you are often snacking on chocolate or eating chocolate desserts, you may want to switch to healthier alternatives like carob, whole fruit and even nut butters which many of may patients love for their creamy, delectable flavor. They will often put nut butters like almond or cashew on banana or apple slices and crackers or muffins for a healthy snack or dessert instead of overindulging on chocolate.

Unsweetened carob tastes like chocolate but is naturally sweeter than chocolate. Chocolate is bitter in its natural state and requires a lot of fatigue and stress worsening sugar to improve the taste. A member of the legume family, carob is high in calcium. You can purchase it in chunk form as a substitute for chocolate candy or as a powder for use in baking or drinks. Be careful, however, not to overindulge; carob, like chocolate, is high in calories and fat. Consider it a treat and a cooking aid for use in small amounts only.

How to Substitute for Sugar

Many women are addicted to sugar, which can worsen fatigue and mood symptoms. Most of us grew up on highly sugared soft drinks, candy, and rich pastries—no wonder the incidence of diabetes is soaring among our population. I have found that as women decrease their sugar intake, most begin to really enjoy the subtle flavors of the foods they eat. There are a number of great sugar substitutes on the market that won't worsen your fatigue and mood symptoms and several even have health benefits. These include:

Substitute healthy sweetening agents. Stevia and xylitol are two of my favorites. Stevia is an herbal sweetener that is calorie free. Thus, it is helpful if you are on a weight loss program or don't want the extra calories found in other sweeteners such as sugar or honey. Because stevia contains no calories from sugar, it does not create imbalances in the blood sugar level. This is very beneficial if you suffer from hypoglycemia or diabetes.

Xylitol is a wonderful sweetener that is derived from woody fibrous plant material. It gives a delicious flavor to baked goods, desserts and beverages without the health problems related to table sugar like diabetes, candida infections, obesity and tooth decay. Even better, xylitol is as sweet as sugar but has only two thirds the calories.

Xylitol is absorbed more slowly than sugar so is helpful for diabetes, has antibacterial and antifungal properties and helps promote healthy teeth and gums. It is also found naturally in guavas, pears, blackberries, raspberries, aloe vera, eggplant, peas, green beans and corn.

Substitute concentrated sweeteners. Concentrated sweeteners such as honey and maple syrup have a sweeter taste per quantity used than table sugar. Using these substitutes will enable you to cut down on the amount of sugar used. If you use a concentrated sweetener in place of sugar in an ordinary recipe, reduce the liquid content in the recipe by one-fourth cup. If no liquid is used in the recipe, add 3 to 5 tablespoons of flour for each three-fourths cup of concentrated sweetener.

Substitute fruit for sugar in pastries. In making muffins and cookies, you may want to try removing sugar altogether and adding extra fruits and nuts. Many of my patients like to use applesauce and bananas as sweeteners in baked goods to cut down the need for sugar.

How to Substitute for Alcohol

Use low-alcohol or nonalcoholic products for drinking or cooking. There are many delicious low-alcohol and nonalcoholic wines and beers for sale in supermarkets and liquor stores. Many of these taste quite good and can be used for meals or at social occasions. In addition, you can substitute low-alcohol or nonalcoholic wine or beer when cooking or preparing sauces and marinades. You will retain much of the flavor that alcohol imparts, and you'll decrease the stress factor substantially.

Use sparkling water for parties and social events. Many of us enjoy holding a beverage while socializing. Instead of alcoholic beverages like wine, hard liquor or a mixed drink, consider sparkling water with a twist of lemon or lime. A splash of bitters is also excellent. Or, combine sparkling water with a little fruit juice for a festive drink.

How to Substitute for Dairy Products

Eliminate or decrease the amount of cheese you use in food preparation and cooking. If you must use cheese in cooking, decrease the amount in the recipe by three-fourths so that it becomes a flavoring or garnish rather than a major source of fat and protein. For example, use one teaspoon of Parmesan cheese on top of a casserole instead of one-half cup.

Use vegan, soy or rice cheese without casein in food preparation and cooking. These nondairy cheeses are all excellent substitutes for cheese. They are all lower in fat and salt, and the fat it does contain isn't saturated.

Health food stores offer many brands that come in different flavors, such as mozzarella, cheddar, American, and jack. The quality of these products keeps improving all the time.

You can use soy, vegan and rice cheeses in sandwiches, salads, pizzas, lasagnas, and casseroles. You can also use small amount of goat or sheep cheese in recipes as they tend to be more digestible and better tolerated than cheeses and other dairy products.

In some recipes you can replace cheese with soft tofu. I have done this often with lasagna, layering the lasagna noodles with tofu and topping with melted soy cheese for a delicious dish. The tofu, which is bland, takes on the taste of the tomato sauce.

Replace milk and yogurt in recipes. For milk, substitute rice, coconut, almond, hempseed, flaxseed, sunflower seed, and soymilk. All of these milks come in various flavors including unsweetened, vanilla, strawberry, chocolate and carob. Three to four glasses of soymilk each day provides a significant amount of the soy isoflavones, which are estrogen-like chemicals that help to regulate mood during the perimenopausal and menopausal years. Soy also helps to regulate cholesterol levels in middle-aged women. Many nondairy milks are good sources of calcium and can be used for drinking, eating, or baking. Soy and nut milks are available at most health food stores.

For yogurt, substitute almond, coconut and soy yogurt. Several excellent brands of nondairy yogurt are available in health food stores in plain, vanilla, and fruit flavors. The taste is excellent and approximates that of yogurt. They are good substitutes for both cooking and baking.

Substitute flaxseed oil for butter. Flaxseed oil is the best substitute for butter I have found. It is a rich, golden oil that looks and tastes quite a bit like butter. It is delicious on anything you would normally top with butter—toast, rice, popcorn, steamed vegetables, or potatoes. Flaxseed oil is extremely high in beneficial omega-3 essential fatty acids—the type of fat that is very healthy for a woman's body. It supports your energy as well as promotes a balanced mood and brain chemistry. Essential fatty acids also improve vitality, enhance circulation, and help promote healthy hormonal function.

Flaxseed oil is quite perishable, however, because it is sensitive to heat and light. You can't cook with it—cook the food first and add the flaxseed oil before serving. Also, be sure to keep it refrigerated. Flaxseed oil has so many health benefits that I highly recommend its use. You can find it in most health food stores.

How to Substitute for Red Meat

Substitute turkey, chicken, eggs, beans, tofu, or seeds in recipes. You can often modify recipes calling for red meat by substituting ground turkey, ground chicken, or tofu. For example, use ground turkey or crumble up tofu to simulate the texture of hamburger and add to recipes like enchiladas, tacos, chili, meatloaf, and ground beef casseroles. Ground turkey and ground chicken are very flavorful. The tofu takes on the flavor of the sauce used in the dish and is indistinguishable from red meat. I often do this when cooking at home.

In addition, many substitute meat products are available in health food stores. These products include tofu hot dogs, hamburgers, bacon, ham, chicken, and turkey. The variety is astounding, and many of these meat substitutes taste remarkably good. The quality of these products has dramatically improved over the years. However, if you are allergic to soy, you should avoid these substitutes and use organic, free range chicken and turkey sausages and hot dogs, free range organic beef or bison hamburgers and other healthier types of meat, instead.

When making salads that call for ham or bacon, such as chef's salad or Cobb salad, substitute turkey bacon and add kidney beans, garbanzo beans, hard boiled eggs, or sunflower seeds. These will provide the needed protein, yet be more healthful and, often, more easily digestible. You can also sprinkle sunflower seeds on top of casseroles for extra protein and essential fatty acids. When making stir-fries substitute turkey, chicken, tofu, almonds, or sprouts for red meat.

How to Substitute for Wheat

Use whole grain non-wheat flour. Substitute whole grain non-wheat flours, such as rice or quinoa flour. These whole grain flours are good sources of essential nutrients, including vitamin B-complex and many minerals. They are also higher in fiber content. These nutrients help to correct estrogen dominance and promote hormonal balance. Unlike the gluten-containing grains like wheat, rye and oats, they do not promote mood related symptoms. Rice flour makes excellent cookies, cakes, and other pastries.

You can also use nut flour and garbanzo bean flour if you want to avoid the use of grain-based flours altogether. These flours can be used to make the most scrumptious and tasty low-carbohydrate breads, pancakes, cakes, cookies and tarts. I especially love using nut flour for my delicious and healthy gluten-free, dairy-free baked goods.

When purchasing flour based products, you can readily find breads, crackers, cookies, cakes, pasta and cereals made from gluten-free grains, nuts and beans. They are available in health food stores, many supermarkets and on the Internet.

How to Substitute for Salt

Substitute potassium-based products for table salt (sodium chloride). Potassium-based products, such as Morton's Salt Substitute, are much healthier and will not aggravate heart disease or hypertension.

Use herbs instead of salt for flavoring. Their flavors are more subtle and will help you appreciate the taste of fresh fruits, vegetables, and meats.

Use powdered seaweeds such as kelp or nori to season vegetables, grains, and salads. They are high in essential iodine and trace elements that support your thyroid health. Hypothyroidism is a common cause of fatigue.

Use liquid flavoring agents with advertised low-sodium content. Low-salt soy sauce and Bragg's Amino Acids, a liquid soybean-based flavoring agent, are delicious when used as salt substitutes in cooking.

Substitutes for Common High-Stress Ingredients

High-Stress Ingredient	Low-Stress Substitute
¾ cup sugar	¾ cup xylitol ½ cup honey ¼ cup molasses ½ cup maple syrup ½ ounce barley malt 1 cup apple butter 2 cups apple juice
1 cup milk	1 cup soy, rice, nut, or grain milk
1 cup yogurt	1 cup soy, rice, or other nondairy yogurt
1 tablespoon butter	1 tablespoon flax oil (must be used raw and unheated)
½ teaspoon salt	1 tablespoon miso ½ teaspoon potassium chloride salt substitute ½ teaspoon Mrs. Dash, Spike ½ teaspoon herbs (basil, tarragon, oregano, etc.)
1 ½ cups cocoa	1 cup powdered carob
1 square chocolate	¾ tablespoon powdered carob
1 tablespoon coffee	1 tablespoon decaffeinated coffee 1 tablespoon Postum, Cafix, or other grain-based coffee substitute
4 ounces wine	4 ounces light wine
8 ounces beer	8 ounces near beer
1 cup white flour	1 cup barley flour (pie crust) 1 cup rice flour (cookies, cakes, breads)
1 cup meat	1 cup beans, tofu ¼ cup seeds

Healthy Food Shopping List

Vegetables

Beets	Eggplant	Radicchio
Bok choy	Garlic	Radishes
Broccoli	Green beans	Rutabagas
Brussels sprouts	Horseradish	Sauerkraut
Cabbage	Kale	Spinach
Carrots	Lettuce	Squash
Cauliflower	Mustard greens	Sweet potatoes
Celery	Okra	Tomatoes
Chard	Onions	Turnips
Cilantro	Parsley	Turnip greens
Collard	Parsnips	Watercress
Cucumbers	Peas (all varieties)	Yams
Dandelion greens	Potatoes	

Legumes

Adzuki
Black
Black-eyed peas
Cannellini
Fava
Garbanzo
Kidney
Lentils
Navy
Red
Soy: tofu, tempi
Turtle beans

Whole Grains

Amaranth
Barley
Brown rice
Buckwheat
Corn
Millet
Oatmeal
Quinoa
Rye

Seeds and Nuts

Almonds
Cashews
Filberts
Flaxseeds
Macadamia
Pecan
Pumpkin seeds
Sesame seeds
Sunflower seeds
Walnuts

Healthy Food Shopping List (continued)

Fruits
Acai berries
Apples
Avocado
Bananas
Berries (like blueberries, raspberries, or strawberries)
Coconuts
Goji berries
Kiwi
Noni
Olives
Pomegranates
Pears
Seasonal fruits

Sweeteners
Brown rice syrup
Honey
Maple syrup
Molasses
Stevia
Xylitol

Beverages
Coconut water
Grain based coffee substitute
Herbal tea
Green tea
Water

Meats
Fish
Free-range poultry
Game meat
Organic lean red meat
Seafood (in moderation)

Oils
Flaxseed
Macadamia
Olive
Safflower
Sesame
Walnut

Foods from Other Cultures
Gomasio
Jicama
Miso
Seaweed (like kelp, dulse, nori, wakane)
Tamari soy sauce
Umeboshi plums

Dairy Substitutes
Hemp milk
Nut milk
Rice milk
Soy milk
Soy, coconut, almond, rice or hemp cheeses, cream cheese, yogurt, and frozen desserts
*Avoid all soy products containing hydrogenated oil.

Herbs & Spices
Basil
Black pepper
Cayenne pepper
Chamomile
Chili pepper, dried
Cilantro
Cinnamon, ground
Cloves
Coriander
Cumin
Dill
Ginger
Licorice
Mustard seeds
Oregano
Peppermint
Poppy
Rosemary
Sage
Tarragon
Thyme
Turmeric

8

Amino Acids, Vitamins, Minerals & Herbs

During my years of working with patients, I have found that the use of therapeutic nutritional supplements can play an essential role in the treatment and prevention of chronic fatigue and depression. They can play an essential role in your own chronic fatigue recovery program. The right mix of nutritional supplements can help boost your immune system, endocrine glands, and digestive tract, and they can help stabilize and balance your mood. They also promote good circulation of blood and oxygen to the entire body, a necessity for high energy and vitality.

When adequate nutritional support is lacking, I have found it very difficult to entirely relieve fatigue. In fact, poor or inadequate nutrition may play a major role in causing fatigue. Numerous research studies done at university centers and hospitals support the importance of nutrition in relieving fatigue.

Even with an excellent diet, it is difficult to take in the therapeutic levels of nutrients needed for optimal healing from chronic fatigue, tiredness and depression. The use of nutritional supplements can help bridge this gap so you feel better as rapidly and completely as possible. I do want to, however, emphasize the importance of a good diet along with the use of supplements. Supplements should never be used as an excuse to continue poor dietary habits. I have found that my patients heal most effectively when they combine a nutrient-rich diet with the right mix of supplements.

This chapter is divided into five sections. The first discusses the role of amino acids in relieving fatigue and depression, the second section explains the beneficial effects of vitamins and minerals; the third section discusses the benefits of fatty acids. The fourth section tells which herbs help relieve chronic fatigue.

Finally, **I conclude the chapter with a chart that summarizes all of the nutritional supplements that I discuss in this chapter as well as recommendations on how to best use nutritional supplements.** I also provide you with a sample nutritional supplement formula and a series of charts that list major food sources for each essential nutrient.

As you read through the chapter, I suggest that you consider using the supplements that are most targeted towards your specific set of symptoms. You may also have specific preferences about the types of supplements that you would like to use. For example, some women are more interested in correcting imbalances in brain chemistry through the use of amino acids while others are drawn more towards using herbs.

I suggest that you begin by using the types of nutritional supplements that you feel most drawn towards that I discuss in this chapter. Vitamins and minerals can often be taken in combination by using a high potency multinutrient product. Nutritional supplements are readily available in health food stores or can be ordered through the Internet.

Remember that all women differ somewhat in their nutritional needs. If you do take the recommended vitamin or herbal supplements, I usually advise that you start with one-fourth to one-half the dose recommended in this book and work your way up slowly to the higher dosage, if needed. You may find that you do best with slightly more or less of certain ingredients.

Amino Acids

In order to ensure you have adequate neurotransmitter levels needed for healthy brain chemistry and hormone production, it can be helpful to supplement with key amino acids, vitamins, and minerals. All neurotransmitters are derived from nutrients that you take in through your diet. They are either produced from amino acids found in the protein that you eat or can be taken as supplements.

If you are interested in using amino acid therapy, you may want to consult with a physician or caregiver who is experienced in using this type of supplementation since it can have significant effects on your brain chemistry and you may want to monitor its use. Certain amino acids help to boost energy levels and combat fatigue. These include the following:

Phenylalanine. Phenylalanine is the precursor of the excitatory neurotransmitters, dopamine and norepinephrine, that I discussed earlier in this book. When you have a phenylalanine deficiency, you are likely to experience fatigue and depression. This essential amino acid must be acquired through diet or can be taken as a supplement. Supplementation with phenylalanine can boost your energy, elevate your mood and provide relief from pain.

In one study, phenylalanine combined with L-deprenyl, a medication used to treat an adrenal hormonal imbalance called Cushing's Disease, decreased the symptoms of depression in 80 to 90 percent of the patients treated. In another study, phenylalanine was found to be as effective as imipramine, an antidepressant drug but provided faster symptom relief. Finally, phenylalanine used alone decreased the symptoms of depression in 74 percent of the patients treated in further research.

Good food sources of phenylalanine include fish, poultry, red meat, soybeans, almonds, lentils, lima beans, chickpeas, and sesame seeds. It can also be taken in purified form as a dietary supplement. Patients on phenylalanine may notice greater alertness and well-being. 500 to 2,000 milligrams per day, taken between meals, is the usual therapeutic dosage. Be sure to start at the lower end of the range, increasing gradually. Phenylalanine is a natural antidepressant and painkiller, but can also cause jitteriness and nervousness when used in too high a dose.

It should be avoided by women using monoamine oxidase (MAO) inhibitor drugs for depression since it can cause an elevation in blood pressure. You should also avoid taking phenylalanine supplements if you have a condition called phenylketonuria. This is a genetic disorder in which your body cannot properly break down phenylalanine. Many soft drinks and other foods contain aspartame, an artificial sweetener that contains phenylalanine. You need to watch your intake of aspartame to avoid overdosing on phenylalanine which can cause headache, nausea and heartburn.

Tyrosine. Like phenylalanine, tyrosine is also a precursor for production of excitatory neurotransmitters, dopamine and norepinephrine, needed for energy, vitality, and zest for life. It combines with iodine within the thyroid gland to form the thyroid hormone thyroxine. Thyroxine controls metabolic rate, promotes growth (particularly crucial in children), and regulates carbohydrate and fat metabolism. It also helps produce melanin, the pigment responsible for our skin and hair color.

Tyrosine deficiency is uncommon. Low levels have been associated with low blood pressure, low body temperature and an underactive thyroid. However, women whose protein intake is low or who can't absorb and assimilate protein due to digestive problems may lack sufficient tyrosine in their diets. These women may have borderline low thyroid levels that can be remedied by increasing their protein intake.

Tyrosine may also be taken as a dietary supplement. Tyrosine can help relieve depression, another cause of chronic fatigue. It has also been shown to relieve some symptoms in patients with Parkinson's disease. The recommended dosage is 500 to 1500 milligrams of pure tyrosine per day, in divided dosages, taken apart from meals. Since tyrosine can increase energy and alertness, it is best to take it earlier in the day so that it does not interfere with sleep. As with phenylalanine, women using monoamine oxidase (MAO) inhibitor drugs for the treatment of depression should avoid taking tyrosine as should women diagnosed with melanoma.

5-HTP. The essential amino acid tryptophan is initially converted into an intermediary substance called 5-hydroxytryptophan (5-HTP), which is then converted into serotonin the major inhibitory neurotransmitter.

While tryptophan is available as a supplement and is abundant in turkey, pumpkin seeds, and almonds, I've found that 5-HTP is a more effective and reliable option for boosting your neurotransmitter production. 5-HTP is very helpful for women suffering from fatigue and tiredness due to sleeplessness and insomnia.

Numerous double-blind studies have shown that 5-HTP is as effective as many of the more common antidepressant drugs and is associated with fewer and much milder side effects. In addition to increasing serotonin levels, 5-HTP triggers an increase in endorphins and other neurotransmitters that are often low in cases of depression.

Diminished serotonin levels are also believed to be a factor in fibromyalgia. In a double-blind, placebo controlled study of fibromyalgia patients published in the *Journal of International Medical Research*, those patients who took 5-HTP experienced significantly less pain, morning stiffness, fatigue, sleep disturbance, and anxiety within 30 days. And, their improvement continued for 90 days before leveling off

I recommend 50–100 mg of 5-HTP three times daily. This nutrient is readily available at most health food stores and online supplement retailers.

To maintain proper serotonin levels, it is helpful to take 50–100 mg of 5-HTP once or twice a day, with one of the dosages taken at bedtime. Be sure to start at 50 mg and increase as necessary. If needed during the day, use carefully, as too much serotonin can interfere with your ability to drive or concentrate.

S-Adenosylmethionine (SAMe). This is a naturally occurring substance that is found in almost every tissue and fluid in the body. It supports immune function and helps to maintain cell membranes. SAMe is important in the production and break down of brain neurotransmitters and hormones, such as serotonin, dopamine and melatonin. Deficiencies of the B vitamins, vitamin B12 and folic acid, may reduce the levels of SAMe in your body. Because of its effect on brain neurotransmitters, SAMe has been found to be helpful in the treatment of depression as well as relieves the pain of osteoarthritis.

Some research studies have found that SAMe is more effective than placebo in treating mild-to-moderate depression and is just as effective as antidepressant medications without the side effects often seen with drug therapy. Another benefit is that SAMe produces therapeutic benefits more quickly than antidepressant medications which can take up to 6 to 8 weeks for their effects to begin. Researchers have also examined SAMe's use in the treatment of fibromyalgia, but the results are mixed. It may be worth a try, however, if you are struggling with the symptoms of fibromyalgia.

The recommended dosage is 800 mg per day. You should avoid using SAMe if you have manic or bipolar disorder or Parkinson's disease. Consult with your doctor if you are taking any mood altering drug about the advisability of using SAMe.

Melatonin. This is a hormone produced from serotonin and secreted by the pineal gland. Its secretion takes place at night and is inhibited by light. As such, it sets and regulates the timing of your body's natural circadian rhythms, such as waking and sleeping. Unfortunately, as you get older, you produce less and less melatonin. This is due, in part, to menopause.

Women who have poor sleep patterns, such as night shift workers, are also more likely to have decreased melatonin production. Drugs such as aspirin, ibuprofen, beta-blockers, calcium channel blocks, sleeping pills and tranquilizer may also deplete melatonin levels.

Melatonin is an essential nighttime hormone that is necessary for rejuvenating sleep. A lack of truly restorative sleep is well recognized to promote fibromyalgia flare-ups and worsen its symptoms. For melatonin to be effective, your bedroom should be dark, as light suppresses its release. Supplementing with melatonin may also be beneficial if you have chronic fatigue due to fibromyalgia, depression, menopause or other causes to improve the quality of your sleep.

To ensure that you have adequate levels of melatonin, I suggest supplementing with 0.3 to 1 mg at bedtime. Paradoxically, less is often better than a higher dosage. In fact, the most effective dosage appears to be 0.3 mg. To help ensure that you sleep through the night, you may want to take melatonin as a time released capsule. However, some women may find that they do better with a higher dosage. In this case, I suggest taking 1.5 – 3 mg.

Vitamins and Minerals for Chronic Fatigue

Many vitamins and minerals are useful in the treatment and prevention of chronic fatigue and depression. While a high-nutrient diet plays an important role in combating fatigue, you may get the best therapeutic results by adding supplements to boost the level of these nutrients. However, if you suffer from chronic fatigue and depression, it is best to start slowly. You may want to begin with as little as one-fourth of the listed dose, to see how you tolerate the supplements. You can then increase your dose gradually until you find the level that works best for you.

While I discuss each vitamin and mineral supplement separately, you will probably be able to take most of them together in a high quality, multinutrient product. Good products are available in health food stores and through the Internet. I provide a sample product formula for you at the end of this chapter.

Vitamin A. This nutrient helps protect the body against invasion by pathogens such as viruses (which might trigger ME/CFS and by bacteria, fungi, and allergies. It does this in several ways. Vitamin A supports the production and maintenance of healthy skin, as well as the mucous membranes that line the mouth, lungs, digestive tract, bladder, and cervix. When these tissues are healthy, invaders have difficulty penetrating the membranes, the body's first line of defense.

Vitamin A also enhances the immune system by increasing T-cell activity (these are important cells that help to fight infectious disease). Vitamin A also contributes to the health of the thymus, a gland located in the chest that plays an important role in maintaining healthy immune function.

Because Vitamin A is needed for normal production of red blood cells, it helps prevent fatigue caused by anemia. It also helps control the tiredness caused by anemia that occurs with heavy menstrual bleeding.

Vitamin A should be used carefully. It is a fat-soluble vitamin that is stored in the body, especially the liver. Dosages up to 5,000 I.U. can usually be handled safely by the body. However, if you choose to take higher dosages, you should be monitored by a physician. An overdose of vitamin A can cause headaches and stress the liver.

Beta-carotene, called provitamin A, is a precursor of vitamin A found in fruits and vegetables. Beta-carotene is water-soluble and, unlike vitamin A, does not accumulate in the body. As a result, it can be used safely in higher doses. Between 5,000 to 25,000 I.U. can be taken as a nutritional supplement. Certain foods, such as sweet potatoes, carrots, winter squash, spinach, kale and collard greens contain large amounts of beta-carotene.

Provitamin A also enhances immune function. It stimulates immune cells called macrophages and helps trigger increased immune activity against certain bacteria as well as candida. Beta-carotene is also a powerful antioxidant that helps to protect the body from damage by free radicals. Free radicals are chemicals that occur as by-products of oxygen use in the body, exposure to ultraviolet light, and other natural processes; they can damage the cell membranes as well as other parts of the cell. Antioxidants like beta-carotene neutralize free radicals.

Vitamin B-Complex. This complex consists of 11 vitamin B factors. The whole complex works together to perform important metabolic functions; including glucose metabolism, stabilization of brain chemistry and inactivation of estrogen. These processes regulate the body's level of energy and vitality. Because B vitamins are water-soluble and are not stored in the body, they are easily lost when a woman is under stress or is eating unhealthy food, including coffee, cola drinks, and other caffeine-containing beverages. Fatigue and depression can result from the depletion of B vitamins. Vitamin B-complex should be included in a nutritional program for fibromyalgia as well as allergies.

Many women with anemia, who are often fatigued, may be deficient in three B-complex vitamins—folic acid, pyridoxine (vitamin B6), and vitamin B12. All three are needed for normal growth and maturation of red blood cells. Their deficiency leads to anemia and fatigue. Supplemental vitamin B12 is necessary for women on a vegetarian diet. It is usually given by injection.

Vitamin B6 is extremely important in relieving and preventing fatigue. In women who are prone to fatigue caused by bacteria, viruses, candida, or allergies, B6 supports a healthy immune response. Vitamin B6 is needed for both the production of antibodies by white blood cells and the production of T-cell lymphocytes by the thymus. This vitamin also appears to help enhance the activity of the T-cells, making them more effective in destroying infectious agents.

Vitamin B6 helps reduce PMS-related mood swings, fatigue, food cravings, and fluid retention through its effect on glucose metabolism and its participation in prostaglandin synthesis. Prostaglandins—hormones that regulate many important physiological functions—are formed in the body from certain essential vegetable and fish oils. The essential fats can only be converted to prostaglandins in the presence of B6 and other essential nutrients. Prostaglandin deficiency adversely affects brain chemistry and mood and can worsen depression and fatigue.

Women using birth control pills and menopausal women on hormonal replacement therapy can be prone to fatigue because the use of hormones causes vitamin B6 deficiency. Finally, B6 deficiency has been found in fatigued women who suffer from depression. Vitamin B6 can be taken safely by most women in doses between 25 to 150 milligrams. Doses above this level should be avoided because B6 can cause toxic symptoms in the nervous system in susceptible women.

The B-complex vitamins are usually found together in beans and whole grains. These foods should be part of the diet of women with chronic fatigue, who would also probably benefit from the use of supplemental vitamin B. I recommend 25 – 100 mg per day of vitamin B-complex.

Vitamin C. This is an extremely important nutrient for fatigue. In one research study done on 411 dentists and their spouses, scientists found a clear relationship between the presence of fatigue and lack of vitamin C. By supporting the immune function, vitamin C helps prevent fatigue caused by infections. It stimulates the production of interferon, a chemical found to prevent the spread of viruses in the body. While it is necessary for healthy white blood cells and their antibody production, vitamin C also helps the body fight bacterial and fungal infections. It is an important nutrient for fibromyalgia and chronic fatigue.

Women with low vitamin C intake also tend to have elevated levels of histamine, a chemical that triggers allergy symptoms. Vitamin C is an important anti-stress vitamin, needed for the production of sufficient adrenal gland hormones. Healthy adrenal function helps prevent fatigue and exhaustion in women who are under physical or emotional stress.

In women with iron deficiency anemia, vitamin C increases the absorption of iron from the digestive tract. Vitamin C has also been tested, along with bioflavonoids, as a treatment for anemia caused by heavy menstrual bleeding—a common cause of fatigue in teenagers and premenopausal women in their forties. Vitamin C reduces bleeding by helping to strengthen capillaries and prevent capillary fragility. One clinical study of vitamin C showed a reduction in bleeding in 87 percent of women taking supplemental amounts of this essential nutrient.

The best sources of vitamin C in nature are fruits and vegetables. It is a water-soluble vitamin, so it is not stored in the body. Thus, women with chronic fatigue should replenish their vitamin C supply daily through a healthy diet and the use of supplements. I recommend 1000 – 3000 mg per day of mineral buffered vitamin C in divided dosages.

Bioflavonoids. These nutrients are found abundantly in flowers and in fruits, particularly oranges, grapefruits, cherries, huckleberries, black-berries, and grape skins. Besides giving pigmentation to plants, they have a number of beneficial physiological effects that can help decrease fatigue symptoms. Bioflavonoids are powerful antioxidants that help protect cells against damage by free radicals. They help protect us from fatigue caused by allergic reactions, because their anti-inflammatory properties help prevent the production and release of compounds such as histamine and leukotriene that promote inflammation.

Bioflavonoids such as quercetin have powerful antiviral properties that protect us from infections. Quercetin also inhibits the release of allergic compounds from mast cells — the cells in the digestive and respiratory tract that release histamine.

Bioflavonoids are among the most important nutrients for mid-life women suffering from menopausal symptoms, including fatigue and depression. Bioflavonoids produce chemical activity similar to estrogen and can be used as an estrogen substitute. Clinical studies have shown that bioflavonoids can help control hot flashes and the psychological symptoms of menopause, including fatigue, irritability, and mood swings. Interestingly, bioflavonoids contain a very low potency of estrogen, much lower than that used in hormonal replacement therapy. As a result, no harmful side effects have been noted with bioflavonoid therapy. I recommend 800 – 2500 mg of bioflavonoids per day.

Soy Isoflavones. These estrogen-like chemicals that are found abundantly in soybeans can help reduce mood swings and depression in perimenopausal and menopausal women. Soy isoflavones are available in capsules and powders. Therapeutic dosages are 50 to 100 mg per day.

Vitamin E. This vitamin can enhance immune antibody response at high levels and has a significant immune stimulation effect. Vitamin E has antihistamine properties and should be used by women who suffer from allergies. One group of volunteers who were injected with histamine showed far less allergic swelling around the injection site when they were pretreated with vitamin E.

Like vitamin C and beta-carotene, vitamin E is an important antioxidant. It protects the cells from the destructive effects of environmental pollutants that can react with the cell membrane. Because it has been found to increase red blood cell survival, it is an important nutrient for the prevention of anemia.

Vitamin E can act as an estrogen substitute. Like bioflavonoids, it has been studied as a treatment for hot flashes and for the psychological symptoms of menopause, including depression and fatigue. It can even relieve vaginal dryness in those women who either can't take or can't tolerate estrogen. According to one study, vitamin E helped skew the progesterone/estrogen ratio in the body toward progesterone. This could be very helpful for women who have heavy menstrual bleeding caused by excess estrogen. Vitamin E is also needed for healthy thyroid function. This is beneficial if you have fatigue and depression due to hypothyroidism.

Vitamin E occurs in abundance in wheat germ, nuts, seeds, and some fruits and vegetables. I recommend 800 – 1600 I.U. of natural vitamin E per day.

Iron. An essential component of red blood cells, iron combines with protein and copper to make hemoglobin, the pigment of the red blood cells. Studies have shown that women with iron deficiency have decreased physical stamina and endurance. Iron deficiency, the main cause of anemia, is common during all phases of a woman's life, because of both poor nutritional habits and regular blood loss through menstruation. Iron deficiency frequently causes fatigue and low energy states.

Women who suffer from heavy menstrual bleeding are more likely to be iron deficient than woman with normal menstrual flow. In fact, some medical studies have found that inadequate iron intake may be a cause of excessive bleeding as well as an effect of the problem. Women who suffer from heavy menstrual bleeding should have their red blood count checked to see if supplemental iron and a high iron diet are necessary.

Good sources of iron include liver, blackstrap molasses, beans and peas, seeds and nuts, and certain fruits and vegetables. The body absorbs and assimilates the heme iron from meat sources, such as liver, much better than the non-heme iron from vegetarian sources. To absorb non-heme iron properly, you must take it with at least 75 milligrams of vitamin C. A standard dosage of iron amino acid chelate is 18 mg per day.

Zinc. Zinc plays an important role in combating fatigue. Supplementation with zinc improves muscle strength and endurance. It reduces fatigue by enhancing immune function, acting as an immune stimulant and triggering the reproduction of lymphocytes when incubated with these cells in a test tube. Zinc is a constituent of many enzymes involved in both metabolism and digestion. It is needed for the proper growth and development of female reproductive organs and for the normal functioning of the male prostate gland. Good food sources of zinc include wheat germ, pumpkin seeds, whole-grain wheat bran, and high protein foods. I recommend 15 – 25 mg of zinc per day.

Magnesium and Malic Acid. Combinations of these two supplements are very important for the maintenance of energy and vitality. Magnesium is required for the production of ATP, the end product of the conversion of food to usable energy by the body's cells. ATP is the universal energy currency that the body uses to run hundreds of thousands of chemical reactions. Malic acid is extracted from apples and is also an important component in the production of ATP.

Magnesium levels are often lower in fibromyalgia patients. In a double-blind, placebo-controlled, crossover study published in the *Journal of Rheumatology*, fibromyalgia patients took a supplement called Super Malic, which contained magnesium as well as vitamin B6, riboflavin, niacin, and malic acid. These patients enjoyed significant reduction in pain, tenderness, and the number and severity of tender points, all within just 48 hours of their first dose.

The recommended dose is six tablets (200 mg of malic acid and 50 mg of magnesium) twice daily. While Super Malic is not currently on the market, these supplements are available either separately or in combination in various products. I recommend starting with a half dose and gradually increasing to full dosage.

Patients with ME/CFS often have low magnesium levels. In a study published in *The Lancet*, 32 such patients were given either a magnesium supplement or a placebo. Twelve of the fifteen patients who received the magnesium reported significant improvements in energy levels, while only one of the 17 receiving the placebo reported a similar result.

Another form of magnesium has been researched for the treatment of fatigue called magnesium aspartate, formed by combining magnesium with aspartic acid. Aspartic acid also plays an important role in the production of energy in the body and helps transport magnesium and potassium into the cells.

Magnesium aspartate, along with potassium aspartate, has been tested in a number of clinical studies and has been shown to dramatically improve energy levels. A fascinating study called "The Housewife Syndrome," published in 1962, enrolled 84 exhausted housewives (who bore a startling resemblance to today's overextended women) and 16 of their equally tired husbands.

After only six weeks of supplementation with potassium and magnesium aspartate, 87 percent of them showed significantly improved energy levels. Similar studies involving almost 4,000 subjects, typically showed improved energy levels after as little as four days of supplementation.

Magnesium is an important nutrient for women with chronic candida infections. A magnesium deficiency can develop from vomiting, diarrhea, and other digestive problems associated with intestinal candida infections. Magnesium deficiency can worsen fatigue, weakness, confusion, and muscle tremors in women with candida infections. Women with these symptoms must replace magnesium with appropriate supplements.

Magnesium deficiency has also been seen in women suffering from PMS-related mood swings, depression and other symptoms. Medical studies have found a reduction in the red blood cell magnesium during the second half of the menstrual cycle in affected women. Magnesium, like vitamin B6, is needed for the production of the beneficial prostaglandin hormones as well as for glucose metabolism.

Magnesium supplements can benefit women with severe emotional stress, anxiety, depression and insomnia. When taken before bedtime, magnesium helps to calm the mood and induce restful sleep. It can also help relieve painful nighttime leg and foot cramps.

Good food sources of magnesium include green leafy vegetables, beans and peas, raw nuts and seeds, tofu, avocados, raisins, dried figs, millet and other grains. I recommend 500 – 750 mg. of magnesium per day. When taken before bedtime, magnesium helps to calm the mood and induce restful sleep. Reduce the dosage if it causes loose bowel movements or on your doctor's advice for other health conditions. You can also take liquid magnesium before bedtime, held under the tongue for two minutes.

Potassium. Like magnesium, potassium has a powerful enhancing effect on energy and vitality. Virtually all of the potassium in your body is inside your cells and has many important roles in the body. Here's just a tiny sampling of the many reasons why too little potassium means not enough energy:

- This essential mineral regulates the transfer of nutrients into the cells and works with sodium to maintain the body's water balance.
- Its role in water balance is important in preventing PMS bloating symptoms.
- Potassium aids proper muscle contraction and transmission of electrochemical impulses.
- It helps maintain nervous system function and a healthy heart rate.
- Potassium stimulates the kidneys to eliminate toxic waste products.

Potassium deficiency has been associated with fatigue and muscular weakness. One study showed that older people who were deficient in potassium had weaker grip strength. Potassium aspartate has been used with magnesium aspartate in a number of studies on chronic fatigue. This combination significantly restored energy levels.

We need at least 4700 mg of potassium each day from our diet, but many of us fall short on our intake. You may also be potassium deficient if you have Crohn's disease, take medications like diuretics, engage in intense athletic workouts or have a very stressful and demanding lifestyle.

Luckily, there are many foods that are great natural sources of potassium. These foods should be included abundantly in your diet and include bananas, almonds, peanuts, leafy green vegetables, avocados, papayas, raisins, citrus fruits and potatoes. Other great food sources include cantaloupe, kiwi, coconut water, tomato sauce, beans, whole grains, yogurt, halibut and salmon.

The negative effect on energy of a diet low in magnesium and potassium is well illustrated by my patient, Kelsey. When Kelsey came to see me she was 45 years old and terrified that exhaustion was going to cost her the life she had worked so hard to create. Until recently, she had been like a house on fire. Her talent, dedication, and willingness to work long hours (many on the road) had allowed her to prosper and buy the home of her dreams—while supporting her mother and two very loved cats.

In the last year, however, something had gone dreadfully wrong. She awoke each day exhausted and foggy-headed. She rallied by 10 a.m., but started declining at 3 p.m., and kept fading until bedtime. She barely had the energy to socialize with friends. She even gave up her favorite pastime, hunting for treasures at the local flea markets.

To try to boost her energy and maintain her productivity at work, she consumed cup after cup of strong coffee with "energy bars," plus what she called "a substantial lunch" (a fast food cheeseburger or fried chicken)—but it wasn't working. Concerned that she might be terribly ill, she consulted her physician, who gave her a clean bill of health when test after test revealed nothing unusual.

But Kelsey knew she was far from fine and was determined to learn why. Fortunately, after a physical exam and taking a medical history and running lab tests, I suspected that her poor dietary habits were to blame. In particular, her diet was virtually devoid of potassium and magnesium.

I came up with a game plan for improving her diet. The coffee, the fast food, and the energy bars would have to go. They would be replaced by more sensible choices, including a wide variety of the magnesium- and potassium-rich foods including fresh fruits and vegetables and whole grains and legumes. I also recommended a nutritional supplement program to fortify her with energy supportive nutrients, including magnesium and potassium aspartate, vitamin C and B-complex vitamins.

Her first follow-up call came a week later. She felt far less tired in the morning, and her energy levels later in the day were noticeably higher and steadier. A month after our initial meetings, a jubilant and vivacious

Kelsey called me to say she was almost her old self and getting closer every day.

Calcium. This mineral helps combat stress, nervous tension, depression and anxiety. An upset emotional state can dramatically worsen fatigue in susceptible women. A calcium deficiency worsens not only mood imbalances but also muscular irritability and cramps. Calcium can be taken at night along with magnesium to calm the mood and induce a restful sleep.

Women with menopause-related depression, mood swings, and fatigue may also find calcium supplementation useful. It has the added benefit of helping prevent bone loss, or osteoporosis, because calcium is a major structural component of bone. Like magnesium and potassium, calcium is essential in the maintenance of regular heartbeat and the healthy transmission of impulses through the nerves. It may also help reduce blood pressure and regulate cholesterol levels and is essential for blood clotting.

Good sources of calcium include green leafy vegetables, salmon (with bones), nuts and seeds, tofu, and blackstrap molasses. I recommend 800 to 1200 mg of supplemental calcium per day. Calcium should be taken with vitamin D and adequate amounts of magnesium for proper absorption and assimilation.

Iodine. This mineral is necessary to prevent fatigue caused by low thyroid function. Iodine, along with the amino acid tyrosine, is necessary for the production of the thyroid hormone, thyroxine. Without adequate thyroid hormone, women may suffer from fatigue, excess weight, constipation, and other symptoms of a slowed metabolism. Iodine deficiency has also been linked to breast disease. Only trace amounts of iodine are needed to maintain its important metabolic effects. Good food sources include fish and shellfish, sea vegetables such as kelp and dulse, and garlic. I recommend 150 mcg of an iodine supplement per day.

Other Beneficial Nutrients for Chronic Fatigue

Digestive Enzymes. Many women with chronic fatigue have poor digestive function. The use of digestive enzymes with each meal can help to improve energy levels. Use pancreatin from animal sources or plant-based digestive enzymes like bromelain (500 mg with meals) or papain (100 mg with meals). These products are readily available at health food stores and through the Internet.

Some products contain a variety of digestive aids, along with enzymes, to help promote healthy absorption and assimilation of food. These products usually contain hydrochloric acid to acidify and digest food in the stomach, ox bile to help emulsify fat and enzymes to help break down fat, carbohydrates, and protein. Plant enzymes such as bromelain and papain digest protein while pancreatic enzymes from animal sources help to break down all types of food. These products may be beneficial if you feel that your digestive function is weak and needs more support.

Take digestive aids with meals and forty-five minutes to one hour after meals are completed. They will help relieve symptoms such as gas, bloating, constipation, and fatigue. If the digestive aid causes heartburn, buy one without hydrochloric acid.

Over-acidity, due to lack of bicarbonate production by the pancreas can worsen fatigue after meals and can create "brain fog." Once the food has been acidified in the stomach, it must be alkalinized by the bicarbonates produced by the pancreas before the food moves into the small intestine. A half teaspoon of sodium bicarbonate, plus 100 to 200 mg of potassium in tablet form one to one and a half hours before a large or heavy meal will provide the buffering so crucial for healthy digestive function. However, consult your doctor if you plan to use an alkalinizing program on a long-term basis, for advisability of use.

Probiotics. These are friendly bacteria like lactobacilli and bifidobacteria that normally colonize the intestinal tract. These bacteria have many beneficial effects on digestion. Because they aid in the production of essential B vitamins as well as acetic and lactic acids, they prevent colonization of the colon by harmful bacteria and yeast. If you have fatigue due, in part, to poor digestive function probiotics are an important part of your recovery program.

Research studies have shown probiotic therapy to be useful for a number of digestive conditions. Certain strains of probiotics have been shown to be helpful for irritable bowel syndrome, Crohn's disease and ulcerative colitis. They appear to help maintain remission in ulcerative colitis and prevent relapse in Crohn's disease. Probiotic therapy has also been found to be very useful for the treatment of diarrhea in children. Research studies have shown that Lactobacillus GG can shorten the length of infectious diarrhea in children and even infants.

If your chronic fatigue is due to candida, it is essential to fortify yourself with probiotics to recolonize your digestive tract with healthy, beneficial organisms. I have worked with numerous patients who have been given antibiotics to treat such common health conditions as bronchitis and urinary tract infections and have consequently developed candida. The vaginal itching, burning, and discharge due to overgrowth of candida in the vagina and intestines then has to be treated as a separate infection.

Beneficial lactobacilli strains are also essential for the health of the vagina and urinary tracts. These healthy bacteria strains normally keep this environment acidic so that harmful pathogens cannot survive. However, a number of factors can throw these systems out of balance. These include the use of antibiotics to treat infections, birth control pills and spermicidal jelly and foam.

Hormonal changes due to menopause can also change the balance of healthy bacteria in the organs and the urinary tract. In addition, the overconsumption of alcohol or sugar and a high-fat diet can reduce the population of beneficial lactobacilli and predispose the body to an overgrowth of harmful bacteria and fungi. Pathogenic organisms like candida may flourish in this environment.

A number of probiotic strains have been researched and been found to be beneficial for women. These strains help to prevent and relieve constipation, gas and bloating and irritable bowel symptoms, which can also occur with fibromyalgia. They help to maintain vaginal, bladder and urinary tract health and thereby prevent infections.

Probiotics also reduce the recirculation of estrogen from the digestive tract, thereby helping to decrease PMS symptoms and other health issues related to estrogen dominance. In addition, they also promote a strong immune system which is important in the recovery from fatigue. Probiotic supplements are readily available in health food stores and through the Internet.

I recommend taking lactobacilli supplements on a regular, daily basis. For maximum effectiveness, take these on an empty stomach, in the morning and one hour before meals. Various probiotics are available as powders, capsules, tablets, and liquids, measured by the amount of viable bacteria per dosage.

For those people who can tolerate dairy products, soured milk products such as buttermilk, yogurt, acidophilus milk, and kefir can also be used to help restore the levels of friendly bacteria. There are also nondairy acidophilus products, such as soy, almond and coconut yogurt, for people who are allergic to dairy foods. Other probiotic-rich foods include sauerkraut and Kimchee.

Colostrum. Colostrum, also known as the pre-milk or first milk, is a form of milk produced by the breast glands of humans and other mammals in late pregnancy. In newborns, colostrum enhances the baby's immune system to provide a lifetime of defense against countless invaders, thereby protecting the infant from disease. There is very good research on the benefits of colostrum protecting infants from acute respiratory illnesses and diarrhea.

It contains many substances that provide benefits for infants including:

- Growth factors, which support growth and healing.
- Antibodies, such as immunoglobulins, that provide protection from invading organisms.
- High levels of protein but lower in fat than ordinary milk. A newborn's underdeveloped intestinal system is not prepared to process fat.
- Acidophilus, a beneficial bacterium that starts colonizing the intestine, helping prevent gastrointestinal infections, including diarrhea.
- Laxative properties that help the baby eliminate meconium, its first bowel movement.

The beauty of colostrum, however, is that its benefits extend to older children and adults as well when used as a supplement from pasture-fed cows. Bovine colostrum, like human colostrum, contains numerous immunoglobulins, which help boost your immune system. Given the issues of antibiotic-resistant bacteria and other pathogens invading our food supply, and the emergence of new and ever more virulent pathogens, the immunoglobulins in colostrum are more important, and more needed, than ever in susceptible individuals. But colostrum also contains other important compounds, such as proline-rich polypeptide (PRP), a substance important in toning down overactive immune systems that may lead to such conditions as fibromyalgia and lupus.

By helping to support and regulate immune function, it can be a beneficial nutrient for healing from chronic fatigue due to fibromyalgia and infection. I have had numerous patients suffering from fatigue for various reasons benefit from using colostrum. One patient, Margaret, who suffered from fatigue, multiple food allergies and inflammatory bowel disease found that colostrum helped to control her symptoms. Joanne suffered from fatigue and frequent respiratory infections found that her energy and immunity were improved when she began to use colostrum.

The recommended dosage for colostrum varies widely, from 400 to 5000 mg, taken 1-2 times per day in capsule, tablet or powder form. You may want to begin with 1000-2000 mg taken 1-2 times per day to monitor its effects and increase the dosage, as needed. You should avoid colostrum, however, if you have a known allergy to dairy products.

Green Foods. I first became interested in green foods like spirulina, chlorella and wild blue-green algae when several of my patients, virtually simultaneously, come to my office very excited about the benefits they were receiving from adding green foods to their diet. These algae are aquatic plants, spiral-shaped, and emerald to blue-green in color, and have been used medicinally for thousands of years in South America and Africa. Many of my female patients who are in their late 30's and 40's have reported that taking green foods helped to lessen the fatigue and mood swings associated with PMS and perimenopausal hormone imbalances.

While I have not found it to be helpful in reducing physical symptoms such as bloating, breast tenderness, and menstrual irregularity, it does seem to promote more efficient liver function. Since the liver has a crucial role in detoxifying and deactivating estrogen, healthy liver function helps to bring estrogen levels back into balance, thereby relieving the fatigue, depression and moodiness often experienced by perimenopausal women. My patients in menopause have also found green foods to be helpful in improving energy, vitality and stamina as well as reducing the symptoms of depression.

Spirulina, chlorella, and wild blue-green algae contain more chlorophyll than any other foods. Chlorophyll helps to neutralize and remove toxins from the body. They are also the highest sources of protein, beta-carotene, and nucleic acids of any animal or plant food, and contain the essential fatty acids omega-3 and gamma linolenic acid. The protein in spirulina and chlorella is so easily digested and absorbed that two or three teaspoons of these microalgae are equivalent to two to three ounces of meat. Further, unlike animal protein, the protein in algae generates a minimum of waste products when it is metabolized, thereby lessening the stress on your liver.

Spirulina detoxifies the kidneys and liver, inhibiting the growth of fungi, bacteria, and yeasts. Because spirulina is so easily digested, it yields quick energy. It is also strongly anti-inflammatory and therefore useful in the treatment of hepatitis, gastritis, and other inflammatory diseases. Spirulina strengthens body tissues and protects the vascular system by lowering blood fat.

Athletes use spirulina for energy and for its cleansing action after strenuous physical exertion, which can stimulate the body to rid itself of toxins. It can also be useful for women who are trying to recover form chronic fatigue. I suggest taking 1 to 2 tablespoons of spirulina, stirred into eight ounces of water per day. Green foods are very concentrated, so start with one teaspoon per day and increase gradually to make sure that it's well tolerated.

Chlorella is a well-known algae that is an especially effective detoxifier and anti-inflammatory agent, thanks to its high chlorophyll content, which stimulates these processes. Chlorella is notable for its tough outer cell walls, which bind with heavy metals, pesticides, and carcinogens such as PCBs (polychlorinated biphenyls) and then carry these toxins out of the body. Because of chlorella's growth factor, this algae also promotes growth and repair of all kinds of tissue.

Chlorella may also help to reduce the symptoms of fibromyalgia. In one study done at the Medical College of Virginia, fibromyalgia patients received 10 grams of Sun Chlorella tablets and 100 ml of Wasaka Gold, a liquid chlorella extract daily for several months. They had significant improvement in fibromyalgia symptoms including reduction of pain.

Take one tablespoon of chlorella in eight to 12 ounces of water. Be sure to begin with a partial dose and increase gradually. The main contra-indication to using chlorella is if you are taking blood thinners like Coumadin since it contains large amounts of vitamin K that can affect clotting.

Wild blue-green algae grow in Klamath Lake in Oregon and are processed by freeze-drying. It is sold under various trade names, frequently as a mail-order product. Wild blue-green algae are very energizing and can improve an individual's mental concentration that can be very helpful if you are suffering from mental symptoms of fatigue.

Try one teaspoon per day as an initial dose and if well tolerated you can gradually increase to one tablespoon of blue-green algae in eight to 12 ounces of water per day. However, do not use in excess since it can cause weakness and a lack of mental focus when used in excess.

Coenzyme Q-10. Coenzyme Q-10 can be a beneficial supplement to take if you are suffering from chronic fatigue. It helps to maximize the amount of energy that can be produced within the body as adenosine triphosphate (ATP), the main energy currency of the body. Coenzyme Q-10 belongs to a family of brightly colored substances called quinones, which occur widely in nature. Good dietary sources of coenzyme Q-10 include whole grains, fish, organ meats, soybean oil, walnuts, and sesame seeds.

It is also produced within our bodies, where it acts as an electron carrier in the energy cycles that take place within the cell that lead to the production of ATP. It is also a powerful antioxidant. Coenzyme Q-10 works in conjunction with vitamin E to scavenge free radicals, thereby protecting the tissues of the body from oxidative damage.

Unfortunately, our production of coenzyme Q-10 diminishes with age, which can have a limiting effect on the amount of energy we are able to produce. Many individuals who are middle-aged and older can benefit from the use of supplemental coenzyme Q-10. Not only does it increase the level of energy production within the body, but it has also been found to act as a mild metabolic stimulant.

When taken at bedtime, it can also be beneficial for fibromyalgia patients by providing muscular, immune and antioxidant support. It is also used by some endurance athletes who may have an increased need for coenzyme Q-10, as well as individuals on anti-aging programs.

Research studies have also found that it improves cardiac function. Its usefulness in treating individuals with heart failure is probably due to its ability to improve energy production within the heart muscle cells. Coenzyme Q-10 has been found to enhance both the pumping and electrical functions of the heart.

The recommended dosage of coenzyme Q-10 ranges from 50 to 100 mg a day. Physicians may recommend that patients with specific health conditions take even higher dosages. Other antioxidants—such as vitamin E, vitamin C, vitamin A (as beta-carotene), selenium, and zinc—should be used in conjunction with coenzyme Q-10.

Caprylic acid. This substance is used for the treatment of candida albicans infections that can occur when the balance between candida and the friendly, beneficial bacteria in the digestive tract is upset. When candida proliferates, it can infect tissues of the digestive tract, vagina and mouth as well as causing symptoms of chronic fatigue, lethargy, depression and difficulty concentrating.

Caprylic acid is a medium-chain fatty acid that is found in coconut and palm oil as well as breast milk. It is an antifungal and is thought to help eliminate candida from the body by breaking down the candida cell membrane, thereby causing a die off of these organisms. A research study published in 2011 found caprylic acid to be superior and less expensive than the antifungal drug Diflucan in its therapeutic effects.

The recommended dosage is 1000-2000 mg per day, taken two to three times a day with meals. It is best to use a timed-release product or as a gel in capsules. That allows caprylic acid to be absorbed gradually throughout the intestinal tract.

You may want to begin with a smaller dose of 500 mg once or twice a day and then gradually increase to the full dosage. Caprylic acid should be taken for two to three months for best results. It is usually well tolerated, although some individuals may experience side-effects like nausea, bloating, belching, heartburn, diarrhea or constipation.

Essential Fatty Acids for Chronic Fatigue

Essential fatty acids help to combat both fatigue and depression so are very important to include in your nutritional supplement program. Essential fatty acids must be taken in through the diet and are the raw materials from which the beneficial hormone-like chemicals called prostaglandins are made.

Beneficial series-1 and series-3 prostaglandins help to create mood and hormone balance within the body. They also have muscle relaxant and blood vessel relaxant properties that can significantly reduce your level of emotional tension and muscle cramps. Additionally, they reduce inflammation within the body. Inflammatory conditions such as food allergies and autoimmune diseases are often aggravated by mood imbalances and stress.

Prostaglandins have a balancing and relaxing effect on the emotions through their beneficial effect on the brain. Taking in sufficient essential fatty acids in the diet can reduce the severity of agitation, sleeplessness, depression and bipolar disorder. Because of their beneficial effects, they have been used in the treatment of PMS, anxiety, eating disorders, and menopause.

Essential fatty acids also help to balance your levels of female hormones and are needed for the production of both estrogen and progesterone during the second half of the menstrual cycle. A healthy balance between these two hormones is necessary to avoid anxiety and fear or depression and sadness since both hormones affect mood.

The essential fatty acids found in fish oil are very beneficial for the relief of fibromyalgia pain. These are docosahexaenoic acid (DHA) and eicosapentanoic acid (EPA) that are found in certain cold water fish like salmon, tuna, mackerel and trout. According to research published in the *Clinical Journal of Pain*, fish oil acts by blocking the voltage-gate channels that transmit signals along pain-sensing neurons. In another study published in the *International Journal of Clinical Pharmacology and Therapeutics*, women with fibromyalgia had significant improvement in pain severity, fatigue, and number of tender points after four weeks of daily treatment with high doses of DHA. To receive this level of benefit, you need to take fish oil supplements that contain at least 2400 of DHA and EPA in combination per day.

There are two main essential types of essential fatty acids that are extremely beneficial for women and help to reduce your vulnerability to fatigue and depression. These are linoleic acid; they belong to the omega-6 family of fatty acids, and alpha-linolenic acid that belongs to the omega-3 family of fatty acids.

Omega-6 is primarily found in raw seeds and nuts. Good sources include flaxseeds, pumpkin seeds, sesame seeds, sunflower seeds and walnuts. Omega-6 fatty acids are converted into the series-1 prostaglandins.

The omega-3 family of essential fatty acids are derived from both animal and plant sources in our diet. These include EPA (eicosapentaenoic acid) and DHA (docosahexaenoic acid) that are found in certain fish such as trout, salmon, tuna and mackerel. Alpha-linolenic acid is found in plant sources like flaxseeds, chia seeds, hemp seed oil and, in smaller amounts, in soy, pumpkin seeds, walnuts and green leafy vegetables. The omega-3 fatty acids are converted into the beneficial series-3 prostaglandins within the body.

Both essential fatty acid families must be derived from dietary sources because they cannot be produced within the body. However, even if the diet contains significant amounts of fatty acids, some women may lack the ability to convert them efficiently to the mood and hormone balancing prostaglandins. This is particularly true of linoleic acid, which must be converted to a chemical called gamma-linolenic acid (GLA) on its way to becoming the beneficial series-1 prostaglandin.

The conversion of linoleic acid to GLA, followed by the chemical steps leading to the creation of the beneficial prostaglandins, requires the presence of magnesium, vitamin B6, zinc, vitamin C, and niacin. Women deficient in these nutrients can't make the chemical conversions effectively.

These nutrients are also needed for the conversion of the omega-3 fatty acids into the series-3 prostaglandins.

In addition, women who eat a high-cholesterol diet, eat processed oils such as mayonnaise, use a great deal of alcohol, or are diabetic may find the fatty acid conversion to the series-1 prostaglandin difficult to achieve. Other factors that impede prostaglandin production include emotional stress, allergies, and eczema. In women with these risk factors, less than 1 percent of linoleic acid may be converted to GLA. The rest of the fatty acids may be used as an energy source, but they will not be able to play a role in relieving anxiety and stress symptoms.

The best plant food sources of the omega-3 essential fatty acids are raw flaxseeds and chia seeds, which contain high levels of both essential fatty acids, alpha-linolenic and linoleic acid. Both the seeds and their pressed oils can be used and should be absolutely fresh and unspoiled. As mentioned earlier, these oils become rancid very easily when exposed to light and air (oxygen), and they need to be packed in special opaque containers and kept in the refrigerator.

My special favorite is fresh flaxseed oil; golden, rich and delicious. It is extremely high in alpha-linolenic and linoleic acids, which comprise approximately 80 percent of its total content. Flax oil has a wonderful flavor and can be used as a butter replacement on foods such as mashed potatoes, rice, air-popped popcorn, steamed broccoli, cauliflower, carrots and bread.

Flax oil (and all other essential oils) should never be heated or used in cooking, as heat affects the special chemical properties of these oils. Instead, add these oils as a flavoring to foods that are already cooked.

Chia seeds are very nutritious edible seeds that were a staple of the Aztec diet. Like flaxseed, they are loaded with beneficial omega-3 fatty acids as well as protein and fiber. Because they are a rich source of alpha-linolenic acid, they can be very beneficial in the treatment of PMS, menopause and other conditions that commonly cause mood symptoms and anxiety.

Chia seeds also have other health benefits. Because omega-3 fatty acids are anti-inflammatory, they help to reduce "false fat" and bloating. They provide relief from other inflammatory conditions including allergies, sinusitis, bronchitis, colds and autoimmune diseases like rheumatoid arthritis and lupus. They also help to regulate your blood sugar level and control diabetes as well as reduce your risk of heart disease

You can eat up to one ounce of chia seeds a day. I recommend sprinkling it into yogurt, oatmeal, smoothies, applesauce or salad or even mix it into your pancake, waffle mix or flour for baking.

EPA and DHA (omega-3 family) are found in abundance in fish oils. The best sources are cold water, high-fat fish such as salmon, tuna, rainbow trout, mackerel, and eel. Fish can be used in your diet once or twice a week but more frequent use of fish should be limited because of the high levels of mercury found in many fish.

Instead, I recommend using mercury-free fish oil capsules as a daily supplement. You should use fish oil supplements, which contain 2000-3000 mg of eicosapentaenoic acid (EPA) and docosahexaenoic acid (DHA). Vegetarians can use algae (seaweed) supplements of DHA and EPA.

My patient, Hannah, had been on a very good nutritional supplement program that had helped to maintain a high level of energy, balanced mood and healthy menstrual cycles. However, she neglected to take her fish oil and ground flaxseeds and other nutritional supplements due to a much busier work schedule while raising her three year old daughter. A few months later, I received a panicky call from her. Her energy had evaporated, she was feeling depressed and was starting to get hot flashes, even though she was only 42 years old. She was distressed that she might be going into an early menopause and needed her normal level of energy to handle her busy life.

After talking with her, it was obvious to me that by stopping her supplements, she was depriving her brain and endocrine glands of the essential nutrients that they needed to function well. Once I explained this to her, she immediately restarted her supplement program, including the fish oil and ground flaxseeds, and she began to feel better almost immediately. Her mood and energy rapidly improved and the hot flashes disappeared! I received a follow-up call from her telling me how thrilled and relieved she was to be feeling so much better.

Linoleic acid (omega-6 family) is found in many seeds and seed oils. Good sources include safflower oil, sunflower oil, corn oil, sesame seed oil, and wheat germ oil. Many women prefer to use fresh raw sesame seeds, sunflower seeds, and wheat germ to obtain the oils.

The average healthy adult requires only four teaspoons per day of the essential oils. However, women with anxiety and stress symptoms who may have a real deficiency of these oils need up to two tablespoons per day until their symptoms improve. Occasionally, these oils may cause diarrhea; if this occurs, use only one teaspoon per day. Women with acne and very oily skin should use them cautiously. For optimal results, be sure to use these oils along with vitamin E.

Herbs for Chronic Fatigue

Many herbs can help relieve the symptoms and treat the causes of chronic fatigue. I have used fatigue-relieving herbs in my practice for many years and many women have found them to be effective remedies. I use them as a form of extended nutrition. They can balance and expand the diet while optimizing nutritional intake. Some herbs provide an additional source of essential nutrients that help boost energy and relieve depression. Other herbs have mild anti-infective and hormonal properties in addition to their nutritional content; these help to combat fatigue-causing viruses and fungi, as well as provide support for the endocrine system with a minimum of side effects.

ME/CFS, Candida Infections, and Allergies

Women with fatigue symptoms caused by severe immune dysfunction may initially have difficulty using any herbs at all because their bodies are too weak. In cases of severe fatigue, I often start the patient on aloe vera and peppermint. Most women can tolerate these two supportive and soothing herbs. You can take aloe vera internally as a juice. Buy the cold-pressed, non-pasteurized brands. You can take peppermint as a tea or herbal tincture in water.

Once you are stronger and less fatigued, you may be able to tolerate herbs that can boost your energy and vitality (see information earlier in this section), as well as herbs that help suppress infections from viruses, candida, and other pathogens.

Garlic is one of the best herbs for this purpose. Garlic contains a chemical called allicin that is a powerful broad-spectrum antibiotic. Studies have shown garlic to be effective against fungi such as candida, as well as the fungus that causes athlete's foot and the dangerous fungus that causes serious cryptococcal meningitis. Garlic also kills bacteria and viruses. In addition, garlic protects the cells through its powerful antioxidant effects.

Echinacea has strong anti-infective properties and can be used to treat pathogens that cause fatigue. It is also a powerful immune stimulant herb. Echinacea helps fight infections by promoting interferon production, as well as activation of the T-lymphocytes (natural killer cells) and neutrophils (the cells that kill bacteria). Native Americans traditionally used this plant as a medicinal agent. I have used echinacea often with patients and have been pleased with its powerful anti-infective properties.

Goldenseal is also an excellent immune stimulant. Goldenseal contains high levels of a chemical called berberine. Berberine activates macrophages (cells that engulf and destroy bacteria, fungi, and viruses). When used in combination with garlic and echinacea, goldenseal is an effective tool for suppressing infections.

Fibromyalgia and Depression

St. John's wort is an herb that has been studied for its mood elevating effects and is enjoying popularity currently as a natural antidepressant. Extracts of St. John's wort, 300 mg standardized to 0.3 hypericin (its active ingredient) have had significant positive effects on depression without the negative side effects usually associated with prescription drugs. It may be used safely three times a day. St. John's wort may also be beneficial for relief of fibromyalgia related symptoms.

For women with fatigue coexisting with depression, other herbs such as **oat straw, ginger, ginkgo biloba, Siberian ginseng and licorice root** (discussed in the previous section) and **dandelion root** may have a stimulatory effect, improving energy and vitality while relieving depression. Women who use these herbs may note an increased ability to handle stress, as well as improved physical and mental capabilities.

The bioflavonoids contained in ginkgo help to combat fatigue by improving circulation to the brain. They also appear to have a strong affinity for the adrenal and thyroid gland and may help to boost function in these essential glands. Oat straw has been used to relieve fatigue and weakness, especially when there is an emotional component.

Insomnia, Irritability and Anxiety

Women suffering from anxiety, irritability and insomnia often have a worsening of their fatigue symptoms because of emotional stress and sleep deprivation. Luckily, a number of herbal remedies relieve such symptoms.

Kava root has been used for centuries in the Pacific islands to encourage a greater sense of well-being and relaxation during ceremonial events. Kava is being used in the West to relieve symptoms of anxiety, stress, restlessness and insomnia. These benefits have been confirmed by clinical studies. The recommended dosage is 140 to 210 mg either one hour before bedtime, or three times a day for anxiety symptoms. Do not use kava for more than 4 to 8 weeks without consulting a physician since it has been linked to some cases of liver damage.

Passionflower has a calming and restful effect on the central nervous system. It has been found to elevate levels of the neurotransmitter serotonin. Serotonin is synthesized from tryptophan, an essential amino acid that has been found in numerous medical studies to initiate sleep and decrease awakening.

Valerian root is also beneficial if you are suffering from insomnia and sleeplessness. Research studies have confirmed the sedative effect of valerian root. I have used it with patients for many years and noted much symptom relief. Other effective herbal treatments for relaxation include chamomile and peppermint teas that also help to relieve stress, indigestion and intestinal gas.

PMS, Menopause and Hypothyroidism

Bioflavonoids. Blueberries, blackberries, huckleberries, and citrus fruit contain bioflavonoids. Bioflavonoids have weak estrogenic activity (1/50,000 the strength of estrogen), but are very effective in controlling such common menopausal symptoms as hot flashes, anxiety, irritability, and fatigue. Plants containing bioflavonoids may be particularly useful for women who cannot take normal supplements because of their concern about the possible strong side effects of the prescription hormones (increased risk of stroke, cancer, etc.).

Other plant sources of female hormones, or plants having hormonal-like effects that are used in traditional herbal medicine, include dong quai, black cohosh, blue cohosh, unicorn root, false unicorn root, fennel, anise, sarsaparilla, and wild yam root. The hormonal activities of these plants have been validated in a number of interesting research studies.

Lower Cortisol and Boost Adrenals

Your adrenal glands produce the stress hormone cortisol. When you are under extreme, chronic stress, your body pours out continual amounts of cortisol. Over time, this excess cortisol can lead to fatigue, weight gain, insomnia, low immune function, and even premature aging. In contrast, low levels of cortisol can indicate that your adrenal glands have become exhausted and are not functioning properly.

Fortunately, DHEA balances the effects of cortisol. In this way, DHEA helps you better deal with all forms of stress, be it physical, mental, or emotional. To this end, many herbs have been shown to improve DHEA levels by helping to lower cortisol and boost adrenal function. I have used these herbs—namely Rhodiola rosea, panax ginseng, Siberian ginseng, and licorice root—as well as the vitamin PABA in my practice for many years, and many of my patients have found them to be effective remedies.

Rhodiola rosea has been used medicinally for nearly 2,000 years. The ancient Greeks revered this rose-like rootstock, as did Siberian healers, who believed that people who drank Rhodiola tea on a regular basis would live to be more than 100 years old.

Rhodiola works to support all hormone production by easing stress and fatigue—both killers of adrenal function and, therefore, healthy sex hormone production, including DHEA. It also appears to stimulate the production of the excitatory neurotransmitters epinephrine and norepinephrine. As a result, rhodiola is beneficial for healing both fatigue and depression.

In one study, patients with mild to moderate depression were divided into three groups, including two groups taking rhodiola rosea and one group who were given a placebo. The participants in the two groups taking Rhodiola reported a reduction in depression-related symptoms like fatigue, mood swings and insomnia with no major side-effects.

Rhodiola is also effective in fighting stress-induced fatigue. In another study, researchers tested 40 male medical students during exam time to determine if the herb positively affected physical fitness, as well as mental well-being and capacity. The students were divided into two groups and given either 50 mg of Rhodiola rosea extract or placebo twice a day for 20 days. Researchers found that those students who took the extract had a significant decrease in mental fatigue and improved psychomotor function, with a 50 percent improvement in neuromotor function. Plus, scores from exams taken immediately after the study showed that the extract group had an average grade of 3.47, as compared to 3.20 for the placebo group.

To ease fatigue, depression, anxiety or stress—all of which can play havoc with your DHEA production—I recommend taking 50–100 mg of Rhodiola rosea three times a day, standardized to three percent rosavins and 0.8 percent salidrosides. While the herb is generally considered safe, some reports have indicated that it may counteract the effects of antiarrhythmic medications. Therefore, if you are currently taking this type of medication, I suggest you discuss the use of Rhodiola rosea with your physician.

Panax ginseng is an ivy-like ground cover originating in the wild, damp woodlands of northern China and Korea. Its use in Chinese herbal medicine dates back more than 4,000 years. In colonial North America, ginseng was a major export product. The wild form is now rare, but panax ginseng is a widely cultivated plant.

Ginseng has a legendary status among herbs. While extravagant claims have been made about its many uses, scientific research has yielded inconsistent results in verifying its therapeutic properties. However, enough good research does exist to demonstrate ginseng's activity, especially when high-quality extracts, standardized for active components, are used.

Ginseng has a balancing, tonic effect on the systems and organs of the body involved in the stress response. It contains at least 13 different saponins, a class of chemicals found in many plants, especially legumes, which take their name from their ability to form a soap-like froth when shaken with water. These compounds (triterpene glycosides) are the most pharmaceutically active constituents of ginseng. Saponins benefit hormone production, as well as cardiovascular function, immunity, and the central nervous system.

During times of stress, the saponins in the ginseng act on the hypothalamus and pituitary glands, increasing the release of adrenocorticotrophin, or ACTH (a hormone produced by the pituitary that promotes the manufacture and secretion of adrenal hormones). As a result, ginseng increases the release of adrenal cortisone and other adrenal hormones, and prevents their depletion from stress.

Other substances associated with the pituitary are also released, such as endorphins. Ginseng is used to prevent adrenal atrophy, which can be a side effect of cortisone drug treatment. Ginseng's ability to support the health and function of the adrenal glands during times of stress, as well as the improved hormone health that occurs with the use of ginseng, clearly supports the production of DHEA itself by the adrenal glands.

In a double-blind study published in *Drugs Under Experimental and Clinical Research*, two groups of volunteers suffering from fatigue due to physical or mental stress were given nutritional supplementation over a 12-week period. One hundred sixty-three volunteers were given a multivitamin and multimineral complex, and 338 volunteers received the same product, plus a standardized Chinese ginseng extract. Once a month, the volunteers were asked to fill out a questionnaire during a scheduled visit with a physician. This questionnaire contained eleven questions that asked them to describe their current level of perceived physical energy, stamina, sense of well-being, libido, and quality of sleep.

While both groups experienced similar improvement in their quality of life by the second visit, the group using the ginseng extract almost doubled their improvement, based on their questionnaire responses, by the third and fourth visits. Thus, ginseng, when added to a multivitamin and multimineral complex, appears to improve many parameters of well-being in individuals experiencing significant physical and emotional stress.

There is also evidence that ACTH (the hormone that stimulates the adrenal cortex) and adrenal hormones, which ginseng stimulates, are known to bind to brain tissue, increasing mental activity during stress.

For maximum benefit, take a high quality preparation, an extract of the main root of a plant that is six to eight years old, standardized for ginsenoside content and ratio. Companies manufacturing ginseng products may mention the age of the plants used in their products as a testimony to their products' quality. Take a 100 mg capsule twice a day. If this is too stimulating, especially before bedtime, take the second dose mid-afternoon, or take only the morning dose. It is best to take either Chinese or American ginseng. Korean red ginseng is too heating for a woman's body and is best used by men.

Siberian ginseng (Eleutherococcus senticosus) has been used in Asia for nearly 2,000 years to combat fatigue and increase endurance. The medicinal properties of this plant have been studied in Russia, with a number of clinical and experimental studies demonstrating that eleutherosides are adaptogenic, increasing resistance to stress and fatigue.

According to a review of clinical trials of more than 2,100 healthy human subjects, ranging in age from 19 to 72, published in *Economic Medicinal Plant Research*, Siberian ginseng reduces activation of the adrenal cortex in response to stress, an action useful in the alarm stage of the fight-or-flight response. It also helps lower blood pressure. In this same study, data indicated that the eleutherosides increased the subjects' ability to withstand adverse physical conditions including heat, noise, motion, an increase in workload, and exercise. There was also improved quality of work under stressful work conditions and improved athletic performance.

Herbalists have also long prescribed Siberian ginseng for ME/CFS. One way in which ginseng may be effective in this capacity is through its ability to facilitate the conversion of fat into energy, in both intense and moderate physical activity, sparing carbohydrates, and postponing the point at which a person may "hit the wall." This occurs when stored glucose is depleted and can no longer serve as a source of energy.

Siberian ginseng is also used to treat a variety of psychological disturbances, including insomnia, hypochondriasis, and various neuroses. The reason this type of ginseng is effective may be its ability to balance stress hormones and neurotransmitters such as epinephrine, serotonin, and dopamine, all of which supports healthy hormone production, including DHEA. Though Siberian ginseng has virtually no toxicity, individuals with fever, hypertonic crisis, or myocardial infarction are advised not to use it. A standard dosage of the dry powdered extract (containing at least one percent eleutheroside F) is 100–200 mg. It is best taken twice a day in the morning and afternoon.

Licorice root has been enjoyed over the centuries as a sweet flavoring for candy and as a delicious tea, but it also has powerful medicinal properties. Its medicinal use has been recorded historically for over 4,000 years. Respected by the ancient Egyptians, licorice was among the treasured items archaeologists discovered (in great quantities) when they opened

King Tut's tomb. Sometime around the year 1600, John Josselyn of Boston listed licorice as one of the "precious herbs" brought from England to colonial America.

Licorice is used to treat respiratory conditions, urinary and kidney problems, fatty liver, hepatitis, the inflammation of arthritis, and ulcers. The herb also exhibits hormone-like activity. Licorice root increases the half-life of cortisol (the adrenal stress hormone), inhibiting the breakdown of adrenal hormones by the liver. As a result, licorice is useful in reversing low cortisol conditions, and in helping the adrenal glands rest and restore their function. This is helpful if you are suffering from chronic fatigue and tiredness.

A standard dosage is 1 to 2 g of powdered root or 450–600 mg in capsule form three times a day with meals. Licorice has activity similar to aldosterone, the adrenal hormone responsible for regulating water and electrolytes within the body. As a result, taking large doses of licorice (10 to 14 g of the crude herb) can lead to high blood pressure, water retention, and sodium and potassium imbalances. Licorice should not be taken by children under age two. Caution should be used with older children, pregnant and nursing women, and people over 65. Start with low dosages and increase the strength only if necessary.

Anemia and Irregular Menstrual Bleeding

Bioflavonoids. Plants that contain bioflavonoids help strengthen capillaries and prevent heavy, irregular menstrual bleeding (menorrhagia), a common bleeding pattern in women approaching menopause. Besides controlling hot flashes, bioflavonoids also help to reduce heavy bleeding. Bioflavonoids are found in many fruits and flowers; excellent sources are citrus fruits, cherries, grapes, and hawthorn berries.

Many medical studies have demonstrated the usefulness of citrus bioflavonoids in treating a variety of other bleeding problems in addition to those related to premenopause, including habitual miscarriage, easy bruising and tuberculosis. Herbs such as yellow dock and pau d'arco are useful for anemia because of their high iron content.

Nutritional Supplements for Women with Chronic Fatigue

Good dietary habits are crucial for control of your chronic fatigue symptoms. But for many women, the use of nutritional supplements is important in order to achieve high levels of the essential nutrients needed to heal chronic fatigue. On the following pages is a sample of the vitamins and minerals as well as their dosages that can be used as a foundation for your program. You can also add the other nutrients like flaxseed oil and fish oil that I have discussed in this chapter to fill out your program.

You may find it easier to implement your program if you start with one of the better quality multinutrient products for women that are available in health food stores and through the Internet and then add the remaining essential nutrients.

Remember that all women differ somewhat in their nutritional needs. If you do take the recommended vitamin or herbal supplements, I usually advise that you start with one-fourth to one-half the dose recommended in this book and work your way up slowly to the higher dosage, if needed. You may find that you do best with slightly more or less of certain ingredients.

I recommend that patients take their supplements with meals or at least a snack. Very rarely, a woman will have a digestive reaction to supplements, such as nausea or indigestion. If this happens, stop all supplements; then resume using them, adding one at a time, until you find the offending nutrient. Eliminate from your program any nutrient to which you have a reaction. If you have any specific questions, ask a health care professional who is knowledgeable about nutrition.

Optimal Formula for Chronic Fatigue

Vitamins

Vitamin A	5000 I.U.
Beta-carotene (provitamin A)	25,000 I.U.
Vitamin B-Complex	
B1 (thiamine)	50-100 mg
B2 (riboflavin)	50-100 mg
B3 (niacinamide)	50-100 mg
B5 (pantothenic acid)	50-200 mg
B6 (pyridoxine)	50-100 mg
B12 (cyanocobalamin)	100 – 750 mcg
Folic acid	400 – 800 mcg
Biotin	400 mcg
Choline	250-500 mg
Inositol	250-500 mg
PABA (para-aminobenzoic acid)	50-100 mg
Vitamin C	2000-5000 mg
Vitamin D	1000 I.U.
Vitamin E (d-alpha tocopherol acetate)	400-800 I.U.

Minerals

Calcium aspartate	500-1000 mg
Magnesium aspartate	250-500 mg
Potassium aspartate	100-200 mg
Iron	18 mg
Chromium	150 mcg
Manganese	5 mg
Selenium	200 mcg
Zinc	15 mg
Copper	2 mg
Iodine	150 mcg

Summary Chart of Vitamins

	Vitamins
Vitamins for ME/CFS	Vitamin A, beta-carotene, vitamin B-complex, vitamin C, bioflavonoids, zinc, potassium, magnesium, calcium, chromium, colostrum, coenzyme C-10
Vitamins for Fibromyalgia	5-hydroxytryptophan, SAMe, melatonin, vitamin B-complex, vitamin C, vitamin D, vitamin E, zinc, magnesium, malic acid, calcium, probiotics, colostrum, green foods including chlorella, coenzyme Q-10, essential fatty acids
Vitamins for Depression	5-hydroxytryptophan, phenylalanine, tyrosine, SAMe, vitamin B-complex, vitamin C, bioflavonoid, soy isoflavones, potassium, magnesium, calcium, green foods, essential fatty acids
Vitamins for PMS	Vitamin B-complex (especially B6), vitamin C, vitamin E, magnesium, potassium, calcium, iodine, probiotics, green foods, essential fatty acids
Vitamins for Menopause	Melatonin, vitamin A, vitamin B-complex, vitamin C, bioflavonoids, vitamin E, soy isoflavones, potassium, magnesium, calcium, chromium, manganese, iodine, probiotics, green foods, coenzyme Q-10, essential fatty acids
Vitamins for Hypothyroidism	Tyrosine, vitamin B-complex including B6, vitamin C, iodine

Summary Chart of Vitamins

	Vitamins
Vitamins for Weak Adrenals	Vitamin B-complex, vitamin C, bioflavonoids, vitamin E, chromium, potassium, magnesium, calcium, digestive enzymes, probiotics, green foods, coenzyme Q-10, essential fatty acids
Vitamins for Candida Infections	Vitamin A, vitamin B-complex, vitamin C, vitamin E, zinc, magnesium, probiotics, colostrum, essential fatty acids, caprylic acid
Vitamins for Allergies	Vitamin A, vitamin B-complex, vitamin C, bioflavonoids, quercetin, vitamin E, digestive aids including enzymes, probiotics, colostrum, essential fatty acids
Vitamins for Anemia	Vitamin A, folic acid, vitamin B12, vitamin B6, vitamin C, vitamin E, iron

Summary Chart of Herbs

	Herbs
Herbs for ME/CFS, Candida Infections and Allergies	Aloe Vera Peppermint Garlic Echinacea Goldenseal
Herbs for Fibromyalgia and Depression	St. John's wort Oat straw Ginger Ginkgo biloba Dandelion root Siberian ginseng
Herbs for Insomnia, Irritability and Anxiety	Kava root Valerian root Passionflower Celery hops Chamomile
Herbs for Menopause, PMS and Hypothyroidism	Dong quai Black cohosh Unicorn root Fennel Anise Sarsaparilla Wild yam root Bioflavonoids from citrus fruits, cherries, grapes and berries
Herbs to Lower Cortisol and Boost Adrenals	Rhodiola rosea Panax ginseng Siberian ginseng Licorice root
Herbs for Anemia and Irregular Menstrual Bleeding	Yellow dock Pau d'arco Bioflavonoids from citrus fruits, cherries, grapes and berries

Food Sources of Vitamin A

Vegetables	*Fruits*	*Meat, poultry, seafood*
Carrots	Apricots	Crab
Carrot juice	Avocado	Halibut
Collard greens	Cantaloupe	Liver—all types
Dandelion greens	Mangoes	Mackerel
Green onions	Papaya	Salmon
Kale	Peaches	Swordfish
Parsley	Persimmons	
Spinach		
Sweet potatoes		
Turnip greens		
Winter squash		

Food Sources of Vitamin B-Complex (including folic acid)

Vegetables	*Legumes*	*Grains*
Alfalfa	Garbanzo beans	Barley
Artichoke	Lentils	Bran
Asparagus	Lima beans	Brown rice
Beets	Pinto beans	Corn Millet
Broccoli	Soybeans	Rice bran
Brussels sprouts		Wheat
Cabbage	*Meat, poultry, seafood*	Wheat germ
Cauliflower	Egg yolks*	
Green beans	Liver*	*Sweeteners*
Kale		Blackstrap molasses
Leeks		
Onions		
Peas		
Romaine lettuce		

Eggs and meat should be from organic, range-free stock fed on pesticide-free food.

Food Sources of Vitamin B6

Grains
Brown rice
Buckwheat flour
Rice bran
Rye flour
Wheat germ
Whole wheat flour

Vegetables
Asparagus
Beet greens
Broccoli
Brussels sprouts
Cauliflower
Green peas
Leeks
Sweet potatoes

Meat, poultry, seafood
Chicken
Salmon
Shrimp
Tuna

Nuts and seeds
Sunflower seeds

Food Sources of Vitamin C

Fruits
Blackberries
Black currants
Cantaloupe
Elderberries
Grapefruit
Grapefruit juice
Guavas
Kiwi fruit
Mangoes
Oranges
Orange juice
Pineapple
Raspberries
Strawberries
Tangerines
Tomatoes

Vegetables and legumes
Asparagus
Black-eyed peas
Broccoli
Brussels sprouts
Cabbage
Cauliflower
Collards
Green onions
Green peas
Kale
Kohlrabi
Parsley
Potatoes
Rutabagas
Sweet pepper
Sweet potatoes
Turnips

Meat, poultry, seafood
Liver—all types
Pheasant
Quail
Salmon

Food Sources of Vitamin E

Vegetables
Asparagus
Cucumber
Green peas
Kale

Nuts and seeds
Almonds
Brazil nuts
Hazelnuts
Peanuts

Meats, poultry, seafood
Haddock
Herring
Mackerel
Lamb
Liver—all types

Oils
Corn
Peanut
Safflower
Sesame
Soybean
Wheat germ

Grains
Brown rice
Millet

Fruits
Mangoes

Food Sources of Essential Fatty Acids

Oils
Flax
Pumpkin
Soybean
Walnut
Safflower

Sunflower
Grape
Corn
Wheat germ
Sesame

Food Sources of Iron

Grains
Bran cereal (All-Bran)
Bran muffin
Millet, dry
Oat flakes
Pasta, whole wheat
Pumpernickel bread
Wheat germ

Legumes
Black beans
Black-eyed peas
Garbanzo beans
Kidney beans
Lentils
Lima beans
Pinto beans
Soybeans
Split peas
Tofu

Vegetables
Beets
Beet greens
Broccoli
Brussels sprouts
Corn
Dandelion greens
Green beans
Kale
Leeks
Spinach
Sweet potatoes
Swiss chard

Fruits
Apple juice
Avocado
Blackberries
Dates, dried
Figs
Prunes, dried
Prune juice
Raisins

Meat, poultry, seafood
Beef liver
Calf's liver
Chicken liver
Clams
Oysters
Sardines
Scallops
Trout

Nuts and seeds
Almonds
Pecans
Pistachios
Sesame butter
Sesame seeds
Sunflower seeds

Food Sources of Calcium

Vegetables and legumes

Artichoke
Black beans
Black-eyed peas
Beet greens
Broccoli
Brussels sprouts
Cabbage
Collards
Eggplant
Garbanzo beans
Green beans
Green onions
Kale
Kidney beans
Leeks
Lentils
Parsley
Parsnips
Pinto beans
Rutabagas
Soybeans
Spinach
Turnips
Watercress

Meat, poultry, seafood

Abalone
Beef
Bluefish
Carp
Crab
Haddock
Herring
Lamb
Lobster
Oysters
Perch
Salmon
Shrimp
Venison

Fruits

Blackberries
Black currants
Boysenberries
Oranges
Pineapple juice
Prunes
Raisins
Rhubarb
Tangerine juice

Grains

Bran
Brown rice
Bulgar wheat
Millet

Food Sources of Magnesium

Vegetables and legumes
Artichoke
Black-eyed peas
Carrot juice
Corn
Green peas
Leeks
Lima beans
Okra
Parsnips
Potatoes
Soybean sprouts
Spinach
Squash
Yams
Snapper
Turkey
Papaya

Meat, poultry, seafood
Beef
Carp
Chicken
Clams
Cod
Crab
Duck
Haddock
Herring
Lamb
Mackerel
Oysters
Salmon
Shrimp
Raisins
Prunes

Nuts and seeds
Almonds
Brazil nuts
Hazelnuts
Peanuts
Pistachios
Pumpkin seeds
Sesame seeds
Walnuts

Fruits
Avocado
Banana
Grapefruit juice
Pineapple juice

Grains
Millet
Brown rice
Wild rice

Food Sources of Potassium

Vegetables and legumes
Artichoke
Asparagus
Black-eyed peas
Beets
Brussels sprouts
Carrot juice
Cauliflower
Corn
Garbanzo beans
Green beans
Kidney beans
Leeks
Lentils
Lima beans
Navy beans
Okra
Parsnips
Peas
Pinto beans
Potatoes
Pumpkin
Soybean sprouts
Spinach
Squash
Yams

Meat, poultry, seafood
Bass
Beef
Carp
Catfish
Chicken
Cod
Duck
Eel
Flatfish
Haddock
Halibut
Herring
Lamb
Lobster
Mackerel
Oysters
Perch
Pike
Salmon
Scallops
Shrimp
Snapper
Trout
Turkey
Raisins

Nuts and seeds
Almonds
Brazil nuts
Chestnuts
Hazelnuts
Macadamia nuts
Peanuts
Pistachios
Pumpkin seeds
Sesame seeds
Sunflower seeds
Walnuts

Fruits
Apricots
Avocado
Banana
Cantaloupe
Currants
Figs
Grapefruit juice
Orange juice
Papaya
Pineapple juice
Prunes

Grains
Brown rice
Millet
Wild rice

Food Sources of Zinc

Grains
Barley
Brown rice
Buckwheat
Corn
Cornmeal
Millet
Oatmeal
Rice bran
Rye bread
Wheat bran
Wheat germ
Wheat berries
Whole wheat bread
Whole wheat flour

Vegetables and Legumes
Black-eyed peas
Cabbage
Carrots
Garbanzo beans
Green peas
Lentils
Lettuce
Lima beans
Onions
Soy flour
Soy meal
Soy protein

Fruits
Apples
Peaches

Meat, Poultry, Seafood
Chicken
Oysters

9

Renewing Your Mind With Love, Peace and Joy

This is one of my favorite chapters in the book because I share with you many wonderful meditations and exercises that you can use to repattern your mind and emotions away from depression and sadness towards a greater sense of love, peace and joy. Even if the cause of your fatigue and low spirits is due to a physical illness, a positive, joyful and optimistic mindset will help to boost your energy and improve your health. A positive mindset helps to balance your brain chemistry and hormones and supports healthy immunity. You can use these exercises in addition to the psychological therapies offered by conventional medicine with great benefit.

Many doctors and psychologists recommend talk therapy and participating in support groups, along with medication, to help manage depression, sadness and low self-esteem. When engaging in talk therapy, you are consulting with mental health professionals in a calm and safe environment. It gives you the opportunity to discuss your feelings of depression, sadness and pessimism that can occur in response to life experiences such as dealing with relationships and events in your life, family patterns and even past traumas.

The goal of therapy is to learn new, more positive ways to respond to the people and issues in your life. This can range from creating behavioral changes, more effective ways to communicate with others as well as developing more positive ways of thinking and feeling.

Your therapist may also help you learn new and more effective ways to manage stress and stress reduction techniques. Some therapists let the client guide the therapeutic process, while acting as a sounding-board or guide to the client's own innate healing process.

Some women find joining a support group of like-minded people who are also dealing with depression to be beneficial. In support groups, the members come together in a sharing and caring environment in which people can openly discuss their personal issues and look to other members of the group for positive support and possible solutions. A support group can be a great place to meet others who are struggling with similar issues.

While talk therapy and support groups can be very beneficial, there is also a great deal that you can do on your own to transform your emotions and repattern your feelings away from depression, sadness and low self-esteem towards joyfulness, positivity and renewed confidence.

In modern times, thousands of studies have been done that give scientific validity to the age-old wisdom that what you do with your mind and emotions has a powerful effect on your health. This is why I advocate focusing your time, attention, and energy on those positive emotions that build you up and enhance the quality of your life and your life force instead of spiraling you down into depression, negativity, fatigue and ill health. These include prayer, love, gratitude, appreciation, laughter and happiness, optimism, a positive self-image, and generosity.

Each of these positive practices and emotions helps to replace and eliminate depression and negativity so that you become a much more joyful, positive and happy person. In this chapter, I share with you many wonderful processes and exercises that you can use to build up and reinforce a strong emotional foundation of positive thoughts and feelings in your mind.

I recommend that you read through this chapter and try the exercises that appeal to you. If you practice them regularly, over time these positive beliefs and emotions will become your main point of focus when interfacing with the world around you.

The Power of Prayer

One of my patients, Laura, shared her wonderful story with me about how prayer and her faith in God finally enabled her to heal from intense defeatism, sadness and depression that were draining her energy and pushing her into a state of fatigue and exhaustion. Laura came into a period in her life when nothing seemed to be working right. She was bored with, and disliked her job. She had a boss who was critical and punitive; and her relationship with the man that she thought he was going to marry broke up in a very negative and acrimonious way. When the relationship ended, she felt very rejected and unloved. She felt defeated by what she called her "dead-end life" and became very tired depressed and sad.

Laura stopped going to social events and seeing her friends. She became more introverted and reclusive. She dealt with her sadness by eating a lot of sweets and other junk foods and gained on an additional twenty pounds to her small frame. Her self-defeating habits further reinforced her feelings of low self-esteem and depleted her energy. Her depression and poor nutritional habits also worsened her symptoms of PMS that became more intense and lasted for up to a week and a half each month; increasing her food cravings, bloating and mood symptoms.

Her best friend, Annie, became very worried about Laura's slide into depression. Annie was a devoted Christian and very strong in her faith. She prayed to God about what she could do to help Laura. She received guidance to go over to Laura's house to visit and pray with her. She did exactly that and asked Laura to read the Bible and pray with her. To Annie's surprise, Laura was willing to do this.

They prayed together for over an hour. During this time, Laura felt God's light enter her and angels lovingly surround her. By the end of the prayer session, she felt that a huge healing had taken place and that God had put her back on the right track with her life again.

Laura told me that she had been totally transformed by this experience. She continued to reinforce her newly found faith by regularly meeting with Annie for prayer and Bible reading as well as attending a church in her community that nurtured and inspired her. Part of her commitment to her healing was to reach out and become more active socially with her friends as well as work with me to get her nutritional habits and body chemistry back in balance and her PMS and fatigue under control. She was able to accomplish these health goals very successfully. Her great faith in, and love for, God continues to guide her life.

Michael's Story

When I first saw Michael, he was in the ICU of the hospital on life support. He had suffered a bleeding episode in his brain and was in very serious condition.

Although his family was living outside of the country, he was blessed by having a large number of devoted friends who constantly visited him and watched over him. Yet, despite being given the best medical care, he continued to be in a very fragile state and remained unconscious.

His doctors finally felt that he had no chance for recovery and were seriously considering taking him off life support. We prayed very hard for a miracle to occur and the next day I received a very excited call from his best friend telling me that Michael had opened his eyes. I rushed over to the hospital and found that not only were his eyes open but he gave me the thumbs up sign as I was leaving his room.

His recovery went very fast from that time on. Even his doctor said that he considered Michael's recovery a true miracle. Michael told me that he remembered all of us praying for him, even though he was unconscious. Tears of gratitude rolled down his face as he expressed his appreciation for our prayers and to God for saving his life and giving him another chance to be with his loved ones, friends and family.

Alicia's Story

I am always inspired by the power of prayer and love! Recently, I was at the hospital visiting with a woman, Alicia, who had been in a car accident. She had broken her pelvic bones and had injuries to her chest and back.

Alicia was in extreme pain, which became worse if she even tried to adjust her position. She was also on oxygen therapy to help her breathe.

Alicia was scheduled for surgery the next day to stabilize her fractured bones, which would greatly lengthen her recovery time. I visited her quite a bit and we prayed together several times. Each time we prayed together, she said that her level of pain diminished.

When I next saw her, I was thrilled to find Alicia lying in bed with a huge smile, surrounded by balloons and flowers and lots of visitors. She had a large family who lived locally and they were all gathered around her and were handling all of the paper work and other details from the hospital. She felt totally loved and nurtured by all of this positive support and attention.

Alicia's recovery was also improving rapidly. Her level of pain had greatly decreased; she was off the oxygen therapy and was breathing much better. Best of all, her doctors had cancelled the surgery, deciding that she could recover very well on supportive care and rehabilitation. She shared with me that she was thrilled to be feeling so much better and felt that the tide had turned with all of the prayers along with the loving and positive support of her family!

Research Confirms the Power of Prayer

Studies from around the world are also confirming the healing power of prayer. One study looked at the cardiac care unit of a hospital in the San Francisco area. Researchers divided the patients into two groups. The patients in the first group were prayed for and those in the second group were not. Researchers found that those people who had prayers said for them had less risk of congestive heart failure and cardiac arrest, and fewer of them needed diuretics and antibiotics, as compared to the group that was not prayed for.

Similarly, a group of 40 AIDS patients were divided into two groups—one that was prayed for 6 days a week for 10 weeks and one that was not prayed for at all. Again, researchers found that the prayed-for group did considerably better than the others. They had significantly fewer new

AIDS-related illnesses, saw their physicians less often, and spent less time in the hospital.

In a study reported in the *Journal of Reproductive Medicine*, researchers tested nearly 200 women who were undergoing in vitro fertilization at a clinic in Seoul, Korea. All were of similar age and had similar fertility concerns. They were divided into two groups. Several prayer groups from the U.S., Canada, and Australia were given photographs of the women in the first group and prayed for the women for four months. Neither the women nor the researchers knew who was being prayed for and who wasn't. At the end of the four months, twice as many women who were prayed for became pregnant as compared to the women in the control group.

In a similar double-blind, placebo-controlled study published in the *American Heart Journal*, researchers divided 150 heart patients (all of whom were scheduled for angioplasty) into five groups. One group received guided imagery therapy, the second had stress relaxation, the third had healing touch, the fourth were prayed for, and the last received no complementary therapy.

The patients, physicians, staff, nor family members knew which patients were being prayed for. After the procedures, those patients who were prayed for had fewer complications than patients in any of the other groups. Researchers were so amazed at the outcome that they have since enrolled over 300 more people for additional studies.

According to a *USA Weekend* poll, more than 75 percent of adults believe that spirituality and prayer can help you recover from an illness or injury, with 56 percent of these same adults saying that they personally have been helped by faith and prayer. And when asked how they felt about having their doctor discuss spirituality, nearly two-thirds felt that it would be a good idea.

But given all this, the reality is that only 10 percent of physicians address spiritual beliefs and needs with their patients. It would be much better to acknowledge the spiritual needs and concerns of our patients to support their healing from illness.

As a physician, I have found that asking patients about their faith helps me understand any emotional and spiritual blocks that might be contributing to their condition and support my patients in their faith. I am also able to learn more about the patients' support network, which helps me to ensure that they have the type of care that will enable them to heal and resume living a full and vital life.

I wrote these spiritually inspired meditations and want to share them with you to support your emotional and mental transformation from depression, fear and worry to faith, hope, peace, joy and inner strength and reinforce your connection to the Divine source of life and goodness.

Love Meditation

- May love, kindness, and compassion fill your heart each day. May you recognize the light of God in everyone close to you and in everyone you encounter in life's journey. May love, kindness, and compassion soften and illuminate your heart, casting a warm glow on the world around you.

- During difficult times, it is important to draw upon your inner strength to help you successfully meet the challenges in your life. Know that you can rely on your inner reserves of courage and self-confidence to help you make the right choices and decisions. At the same time, you need to be flexible in your approach, willing to change course, and allow yourself to find new and even better solutions when confronted with road blocks or challenges.

- Remember that each day is a fresh beginning. Your life, health, and sense of well-being benefits immeasurably when you live each day joyfully, filled with the positive expectations of the many good things that flow to you. It is with this positive attitude that you align yourself with Divine light and love.

I want to share with you one of my favorite meditations. It is a beautiful meditation on filling yourself with the Divine light and love of God. This meditation will also help you release any tension or negativity from your mind and fill you with wonderful feelings of peace and joy.

Divine Light Meditation

- Begin the meditation by finding a quiet place. It can be a peaceful room in your house or office or even a beautiful spot in your backyard.

- Then, sit or lie in a comfortable position, with your arms resting gently by your sides.

- Close your eyes and breathe deeply. Let your breathing be slow and relaxed.

- Visualize yourself as a flower in the sun, opening yourself to God's light and love. Feel this Divine light surrounding you and enfolding you, filling every cell of your body with love.

- As this light fills and nurtures you, you are being cleansed of all cares and worries. This Divine light is dispelling all darkness as it gently and lovingly restores you to a state of health, balance and peace.

- Visualize this Divine light, bringing brightness and clarity into your mind, your head and then your neck and shoulders. As it moves through you, it carries away any tension and tightness.

- Feel the warmth of this light as it moves into your chest and down your arms and hands, and then into your abdomen, bringing with it healing and protection.

- Next, let this Divine light move into your hips and pelvis and finally down into your legs and feet.

- Let this Divine light move through you as long as you would like it to. Continue this process until you feel totally at peace and deeply relaxed.

- Know that God is always with you, caring for you and loving you always.

Love - The Great Healer

At the deepest spiritual and emotional level, our purpose in life is to express our love and appreciation for ourselves, our family, friends, co-workers, and the entire world and all of God's creatures that we share this world with. Love has tremendous healing power and can enable us to overcome stress and fatigue better than any other emotion. When you connect with the love that lies within your heart and express it often to those around you, you will be positively transformed. It allows us to reach out beyond our own concerns and upsets and focus on loving and caring for others. There is also no other emotion that is more immensely self-nurturing and self-healing.

As a physician, I have seen the healing power of love many times. I have always been touched by the great care and acts of helpfulness that many of my women patients show to their children, spouses, other family members, and friends when they're ill. It has always heartened me to see families gather together and support a loved one who is ailing.

I have found that people tend to heal much faster and more completely when they're supported by love and caring. This is not just my own belief; many studies attest to the importance of love and positive relationships in creating health and wellness.

Conversely, I have seen feelings of depression, fear and other intense negative emotions literally wreak havoc on patients' physical and chemical well-being. Many patients I work with have themselves linked their poor immunity, menstrual disorders, digestive upset, high blood pressure, aching joints, and a host of other ailments to the negative and upsetting emotions they were feeling at the time. Many research studies also confirm the negative health effects that emotions like anger, depression, and loneliness cause. These studies find social isolation and lack of close relationships—the inability to connect with others in a loving way—also increases the likelihood of illness. Cultivating your love, caring and compassion are the greatest antidotes for all of these issues.

Follow Your Heart

Follow your heart in everything you do. It is important to make all of your choices out of love, kindness, and joy. These heartfelt emotions are just as important in making decisions about your life as the logical arguments and rationalizations generated by your mind. It is the love that is centered in your heart that responds to the deepest yearnings of your soul—enabling you to create a happy and meaningful life.

The crucial role your heart plays in creating your consciousness differs from the principles of conventional Western medicine, which greatly favors your brain. However, the ancient wisdom found in our spiritual traditions deems the heart as the seat of the consciousness beyond the mind. Much fascinating medical and scientific research is now confirming this connection. There are many wonderful verses on the importance of our hearts in blessing our lives in the Bible. Here are a few of these inspiring:

1 Samuel 16:7 "Man looks at the outward appearance, but the Lord looks at the heart."

Psalm 19:8 "The precepts of the Lord are right, giving joy to the heart. The commands of the Lord are radiant, giving light to the eyes."

Psalm 51:10 "Create in me a pure heart, O God, and renew a steadfast spirit within me."

Proverbs 15:30 "A cheerful look brings joy to the heart, and good news gives health to the bones. "

Mathew 5:8 "Blessed are the pure in heart for they will see God."

Mark 12:30 "Love the Lord your God with all your heart and with all your soul and with all your mind and with all your strength....and to love your neighbor as yourself."

Thoughts on Love

I want to share these heartfelt thoughts about love with you. When you do any meditations, find a quiet place where you can sit comfortably. Close your eyes, and let your arms rest easily at your side. As you take a deep breath, focus on the area of your heart (located just to the left of the center of your chest).

At One With Life

No matter where love comes from or how it manifests, it is important for you to remember who you are. You are a beloved child of God

Feeling Love

Focus on the people and things in your life that you love. Perhaps it is your children, your significant other or your best friend. Maybe you love your faithful dog or cat or even your favorite garden. Focus on how all of these beloved things make you feel. Enjoy the feelings of warmth and happiness that come from focusing on love.

Accepting Love

For many women, the giving of love is easier than the accepting of love. Love can be tied to vulnerability and, if you are struggling with stress and depression, what a scary place this can be. It is important to remember that love itself cannot harm you. True love is patient, generous, compassionate and kind

Loving Visualization

I want to share a loving visualization with you. It is meant to give you a few minutes to turn inward and get back in touch with loving yourself through self-nurturance. This will help you release any negative thoughts or upsets you may have accumulated throughout the day and help you reconnect with the healing power of love.

To do this visualization, find a quiet spot where you can sit or lie comfortably. As you take a deep breath, focus on the area of your heart (located just to the left of the center of your chest).

- As you inhale and exhale slowly and deeply, close your eyes and envision your heart as a luminous, emerald green jewel glowing with love and sending out brilliant light from behind your breastbone, where your heart resides.

- As you breathe slowly, begin to fill your heart with love. Feel the area surrounding your heart soften and expand as you fill it with loving and peaceful energy.

- Then, send love and appreciation to every part of your body, even the parts that you are concerned about or feel are less than lovable. They are all parts of you and worthy of the deepest love and caring.

- Breathe love and appreciation into your head, neck, shoulders, chest and down your arms and hands.

- Send this loving and healing breath next into your abdomen, hips, legs and feet.

- Continue loving and appreciating yourself until you feel your entire body overflowing with love.

- Now, gently open your eyes and slowly begin to move around again. Enjoy the feelings of love, peace and gratitude you have created.

Embrace Gratitude and Appreciation

As a healer, I have been very impressed by how much feelings of gratitude and appreciation have greatly reduced the level of depression, isolation and improved the energy, health, and well-being of many of my patients over the years. These are positive qualities that I always strive to find in myself and express to everyone around me on a daily basis.

However, I did not discover any real research that had been done in this area until the some years ago. At that time, I was introduced to the innovative and groundbreaking work that was taking place at the Institute of HeartMath (IHM) in Boulder Creek, California.

Early one morning I received a call from a medical laboratory that wanted to introduce me to their facilities and services. In the course of the conversation, they told me about very exciting research they were doing with the Institute. Specifically, laboratory testing was confirming that individuals who used techniques developed by the Institute to help them alleviate their feelings of anger, stress and upset, and convert these emotions into feelings of gratitude and appreciation, were having dramatic improvements in several important chemical indicators of good health. From a medical perspective, these findings had amazing implications.

I was so intrigued by the work being done at the Institute that I called and requested their literature and research studies. After carefully reading their findings and conclusions, I was even more convinced of what I had been observing with my patients and myself—that there is a very strong, medically sound connection between positive emotions, such as gratitude, and good health.

The researchers at the IHM found that the heart plays a far more central role in stress, mental and emotional balance, and perception than previously thought. They found that the heart initiates most of the repetitious patterns within the body, and has a much more intricate communication pattern with the brain than does any other major organ.

Plus, the heart not only responds to any stimulus the brain processes—from thoughts and emotions to light and sound—it also generates many times more electrical power than the brain. The signal is so strong that the current sent out by the heart radiates throughout the body. For all these reasons, the heart is in a unique position to connect the mind, body, and spirit.

To test this theory, researchers fed two groups of rabbits a diet that was high in fat. Rabbits from the first group were held, petted, and talked to, while those in the other group were treated normally and were not shown any affection. Interestingly, they found that the rabbits that had been treated lovingly developed significantly less atherosclerosis than those rabbits that had not.

Based on this and other research, the IHM developed specific techniques to stop negative thoughts that would normally engender fear and worry and convert them to positive feelings or emotions. By learning to generate feelings of sincere love, gratitude, and appreciation, a person's pulse, respiration, and brain wave frequencies are better able to synchronize.

In order to examine the health benefits of these techniques, the researchers then did a series of fascinating studies in which they taught these techniques to volunteers, then measured changes in various physical and chemical parameters. The results were very promising, as volunteers had more harmonious and efficient functioning of their cardiovascular, immune, and hormonal systems.

Most telling is that the people who have become adept at using these techniques have reported dramatic increases in the ability to solve problems and handle stresses such as conflicts on the job, rush hour traffic, and rebellious children.

The IHM found that appreciation can significantly increase your body's production of the steroid hormone DHEA. This is particularly exciting for women wanting to improve their hormonal health and balance. Researchers took DHEA samples from 28 volunteers, then asked them to listen to music specifically designed to promote a sense of peacefulness and emotional balance every day for one month.

At the end of the month, researchers took a second DHEA sample from the volunteers. The results were impressive. Among all volunteers, DHEA levels increased, on average, 100 percent; for some, the levels tripled and even quadrupled. This is extremely important for female hormonal balance, since DHEA is converted within your body to estrogen and testosterone.

In addition, the researchers found that feelings of care and appreciation can boost levels of an immune antibody called IgA, which is an important part of your body's defense against bacteria and viruses. And while anger is known to suppress your immune system, they discovered that even remembering a previous angry experience had a negative, long-term impact on immune function.

Conventional Medicine Weighs In

Interestingly, the *American Journal of Cardiology* also featured a study that found that gratitude and appreciation might be positively associated with a reduction in blood pressure. However, it was several years before another mainstream medical journal would present additional support for the Institute of HeartMath's findings.

In a study from the *Journal of Social and Clinical Psychology*, researchers divided volunteers into three groups. The first group kept a daily log of five complaints, the second group wrote down a daily list of five things they were better at/did better than their peers, and the third group kept a daily log of five things they were grateful for. After three weeks, those who kept the gratitude journal reported increased energy, less health complaints, and greater feelings of overall well-being as compared to the participants in the other two groups.

This finding was corroborated in the *Journal of Personality and Social Psychology* when researchers found that many of their subjects used gratitude as a positive way to cope with acute and chronic life stressors.

Express Your Gratitude

Journaling is a fantastic way to express your feelings of gratitude and appreciation. In her book Simple Abundance, author Sarah Ban Breathnach talks about a "gratitude journal." She recommends that you write down at least five things each day that you are thankful for, thereby forcing you to focus on what is going right in your life rather than what is going wrong. I couldn't agree with her more. Regardless of the type of journal you choose to keep, there are a few things to keep in mind:

- Select any kind of journal you want. Some women have used spiral notebooks, others a loose-leaf notebook, still others a gold-trimmed, bound book. What you choose is up to you.

- Make an appointment with yourself for fifteen minutes to half an hour each day to write.

- Choose a safe, calming location where you can write freely, without being disturbed.

- Do not censor yourself as you write - write down your emotions, good and bad. Once the thoughts and feelings are on paper, you can always throw them out if you choose to. The important thing is to get them out.

- Do not worry about punctuation or grammar.

- Finally, be free, be honest, be candid—be yourself.

Similarly, one of my favorite books is *The Art of Thank You: Crafting Notes of Gratitude* (Beyond Words Publishing, Inc.). This beautiful book suggests sending thank you notes as a way to show generosity, gratitude, and kindness to others. Why not show the same consideration to yourself? Why not start each day thanking and appreciating your body? Your family and friends?

Write these positive thank you's and appreciative thoughts as affirmations in your journal, say them out loud in the privacy of your bedroom or office, or even visualize sending loving messages to your body each day. Over time, releasing more and more of your own toxic emotions and replacing them with kind and loving thoughts to yourself will help to diminish the load on your body, mind, and spirit. Then your body will begin to be filled with the most wonderful light, radiance, and health.

Love and Gratitude Meditation

This is a great meditation to do to help you reconnect with the healing power of love, forgiveness, and gratitude.

1. Find a quiet spot where you can sit or lie comfortably.

2. Close your eyes, and let your arms rest easily at your side. As you take a deep breath, focus on the area of your heart (located just to the left of the center of your chest).

3. As you slowly inhale and exhale, imagine you're filling your heart with love. Feel the area surrounding your heart soften and expand as you fill it with loving and peaceful energy.

4. Now, direct your breath into all of the parts of your body, starting with your feet and moving up through your body, finally into your head and neck.

Notice any areas where you have stored any negative or upsetting emotions such as frustration, anger, or other feelings that make certain parts of your body feel tense, tight, heavy, or devitalized.

Keep breathing love into those parts of your body until they, too, relax and soften. By the time you're done, you should feel much more quiet and peaceful.

5. Now visualize your love radiating out from you and touching everyone you love and care about. If you choose to, you can send your love and the spirit of healing to your community, to our country, and even the entire earth.

6. Now gently open your eyes and slowly begin to move around again. Enjoy the feelings of love, peace, and gratitude you have created.

Practice Forgiveness

Practicing forgiveness of others is essential to transforming depression and stress into a greater sense of peace, calm and joy. In my practice, I've seen conditions as diverse as heart disease, high blood pressure, arthritis, inflammation, allergies, and immune disorders aggravated by frequent and constant feelings of resentment and anger. I've also seen unresolved and unexpressed anger contribute to menstrual problems, excessive weight gain and a host of other physical ailments.

In fact, several studies have also linked anger to neck and backaches, muscle tension, elevated homocysteine levels, and increased progression of coronary atherosclerosis. If you too suffer from unresolved anger and illnesses that can result from keeping it bottled up inside, then take heart. It is possible for you to release the offensive feelings and move forward with your life.

Erin's Story

I was recently chatting with my friend Erin who shared with me that anger was the one emotion she was always afraid to express. Several decades ago, Erin's mother and aunt had a major disagreement. They didn't speak to one another for years, and never had the opportunity to reconcile before the aunt's death.

Over time, Erin began to equate expressing anger or upset with a loss of love or friendship. As a result, she has held in any resentment or frustration she has felt toward those close to her rather than express her feelings to her family or friends. The idea of expressing her angry and upsetting feelings and losing love as a result made her feel constantly anxious and fearful.

The irony is that the only one affected was Erin. The people she was angry with went about their daily lives completely unaffected and unaware of Erin's anxiety and stress over her unexpressed upset In addition, her anxiety caused worsening hot flashes, chronic headaches, digestive upset and emotional paralysis. As Erin finally began to forgive the people she had so much upset with, let go of her anger and start to express her emotions, her feelings of anxiety began to diminish and her physical symptoms began to ease up.

Strange as it may sound, many women are hesitant to let go of their anger and resentment. Not only is it hard for many of us to forgive others, but it is difficult to forgive ourselves for our own personal faults and weaknesses. Frequently, anger becomes a comfortable, familiar barrier between you and disappointment or upset. But trust me when I tell you that the only way for good, positive changes to come into your life is for you to take action now to forgive the person who wronged you, forgive yourself, and move on.

Once you empower yourself to take charge of and responsibility for your emotional responses, the rewards will come pouring in. You may reconcile and heal relationships that have been tainted by resentment, anger, and pain. Marriages, families, and friendships that have been strained for years may improve. You could lose unwanted weight or lessen the frequency of debilitating headaches. But most importantly, your quality of life will drastically improve, providing you with greater peace, contentment, and optimism in your life and in your relationships.

If you have a problem dealing with or letting go of resentment, anger, and pain—and forgiving yourself and those you perceive as having hurt you—here are a few suggestions to help you start turning that pattern around quickly and effectively:

1. When you feel upset, learn to express your feelings quickly, in a way that allows you to find positive solutions to your grievances. This will help you to resolve situations that you may have felt stuck in for years, and regain more hope and joy in your life with all of your relationships. Then learn to focus on your appreciation of others, rather than on what angers or upsets you.

2. The most powerful antidotes to anger are the words "I forgive you," "I appreciate you," and "thank you." Learn to say and feel these words often to the people and situations in your life.

3. Look at the positive aspects of your life rather than feeling angry and resentful for what you feel you don't have or what you lack. This will also help you to heal long-standing hurts.

4. If your relationships with certain people or situations turn out to be unworkable and only trigger anger and upset rather than happiness or pleasure, consider gently and lovingly letting them go from your life rather than staying stuck in constant anger or upset.

Change the Anger to Appreciation

The following affirmations take about one minute to do, but can have lifelong benefits. Keep them nearby and repeat them any time you feel anger and resentment building up inside of you.

1. I enjoy focusing on and giving thanks for all of the many positive people and situations in my life.

2. When people or situations cause me to feel upset, I look for positive ways to deal with my grievances so that I feel pleased with the outcome.

3. I seek to deal with the upsets and challenges in my life with a sense of calm and peacefulness.

4. I communicate my feelings of anger and upset when necessary in a kind and thoughtful way that will do no harm to myself or others.

5. I let go of resentment and don't allow it to accumulate inside of me.

6. I enjoy finding new ways to make my life even more positive and joyful.

7. I forgive all of those people who have caused me to feel upset and angry in the past.

8. I forgive myself.

A Blessing for Appreciation

Each day, it is very beneficial to take your focus off of fear, worry and hopelessness and instead give appreciation to those you love and cherish. I recommend sharing the following words of gratitude:

- Thank you for being there for me.

- Thank you for caring.

- Thank you for listening to me during my times of need.

- Thank you for your kind touch.

- Thank you for your love.

Live for Laughter

I absolutely love to laugh and always enjoy finding the fun and lightness in every situation that I can in my life. I think it's one of the most powerful and effective healing tools there are. There is no doubt that positive emotions like laughter and joy have tremendous health benefits—plus, they make your life more wondrous and enjoyable.

I have found that boosting your daily laughter is a great way to transform depression into joy and relax the tensions we are holding. That's why I developed the stress-to-laughter index. It comes from observing the stories my patients have shared with me over the years, as well as examining my own life and those of my friends and family. And what I've seen is that this index can really help you judge how effectively you are providing stress relief for yourself.

If you have too much depression, emotional pain, heaviness, seriousness or concerns and not enough fun and laughter in your life, it's time to flip the scales in the other direction. I've seen thousands of cases of patients getting flare-ups of illnesses, such as colds, flus, immune breakdowns, worsening of menopause symptoms, menstrual cramps, PMS, and painful arthritic episodes immediately following periods of too much stress and heaviness in their lives.

Often, just by flipping into a state of laughter and fun, you can help to bring yourself back into a state of optimal health. Depression and sadness are diminished, your immune system functions better, your hormones are more likely to be in balance, and pain is reduced when you laugh and have fun, thanks to a whole cascade of positive chemicals within your body that are released during times of joy and fun.

To this point, I can distinctly remember a time I was working too much and was feeling a lot of worry and pressure over meeting deadlines. I noticed that it began to have negative effects on my body. I was waking up in the morning feeling stiff, my neck was tense, and my muscles were tight. I also noticed that I wasn't digesting my food quite as well. In short, I was pushing myself to a place of too much stress. I quickly realized that it was time for me to give myself a big dose of laughter, fun, and pleasure to bring myself into healthy balance.

I decided to take a break from my busy routine and take my daughter to the local toy store and have some fun. We bought paint, drawing materials, puzzles and other toys. When we came home, we laid our treasures out on the dining room table, then spent the entire evening playing with our paints, toys and games. It was definitely the right antidote for me and helped me release my tension and stress over my work deadlines and get back into balance.

I noticed that with all of the joy and laughter, my muscles started to loosen up and feel better. The next morning, I woke up and felt much more refreshed, light, and energetic. I even found that I was digesting my food normally again. In short, laughter truly is the best medicine.

Mainstream Medicine Has a Sense of Humor

The healing power of laughter has been the subject of many studies. According to an article published in *Family Practice News*, children laugh, on average, about 400 times a day, while adults only laugh about 15 times a day. This is a sad state of affairs, because when laughter is your automatic response to stress, trying times are less likely to feel anxious and fearful.

Dr. Norman Cousins introduced this concept to medicine after he was diagnosed with a severe health condition called ankylosing spondylitis. He was determined to find a treatment for his disabling condition, and essentially cured himself by listening to recordings of laughter, watching lots of funny movies, and taking large doses of vitamin C.

More recently, research studies have provided scientific confirmation of this phenomenon. Laughter has been shown to lower the stress hormone cortisol, as well as blood pressure and heart rate, and to increase mood-elevating beta-endorphins—natural, feel-good chemicals produced by your body that are 200 times more potent than morphine.

And when it comes to smiles, it turns out they really are contagious. Researchers at the University of California at San Francisco determined that there are 19 different kinds of smiles, all of which are extremely contagious! In addition, Russian research has found that frequent smiling helps people heal from a host of degenerative diseases.

Whatever your sense of humor calls for, indulge it. Go on a laughter odyssey and discover what tickles your funny bone. Whether you like to watch silly movies, read funny books, tell or listen to jokes, visit a comedy club, play games, or go to the toy store, I strongly recommend that you enjoy a little levity as often as possible. And always try to see the humor in the little frustrations and minor disasters that occur every day. It can greatly improve the quality of your life, and just might even save it!

Hold on to Happiness

Your state of health is very closely tied to how truly happy you are. A study on this important subject, published in the *Proceedings of the National Academy of Sciences*, found that people who consider themselves happy are more likely to be healthy and resistant to disease. They also have lower levels of the stress hormone cortisol and a reduced risk of heart disease. This study joins an ever-growing body of research that proves the importance of creating a life in which positive feelings of love, happiness, joy, and optimism predominate over negativity.

There is one particular study I love. Researchers studied the longevity of a group of 178 Catholic nuns from a convent in Milwaukee. The nuns lived together and taught in the same school. They had the same daily routine, ate the same food, didn't smoke or drink alcohol, had the same financial situation, and had identical medical care.

The researchers then looked at the writings each nun did prior to taking her vows. A separate team of psychologists then assessed the positive and negative comments made in the writings, and divided the sisters into different classifications based on the degree of joy and satisfaction in their letters.

The researchers then took these classifications and matched them against the life spans of each of the nuns. They found that 90 percent of those nuns who fell into the "most happy" category were still alive at 85 years old. Conversely, only 34 percent of those who were categorized as "least happy" lived to be 85.

Other studies have shown comparable results. A two-year study of 2,000 people over the age of 65 found that the mortality rate of those people who expressed the most negative emotions was twice as high as those who expressed positive emotions. Similarly, a study from Finland discovered that of the 96,000 widowed people surveyed, the surviving spouse's risk of dying doubled in the week following their spouse's death.

Attributes of Happy People

In the following list, I share many attributes of happy people. If you don't recognize yourself in at least three or four, aim to practice these principles so you can become "One of the Happiest People You Know."

1. Appreciate the many blessings that you already have in your life. When you focus on the positives in your life, it will draw even more to you!

2. Find something to love, appreciate and admire about everyone—and everything—in your life. Have a genuine sense of self-worth and always look for the good in others.

3. Know that you can choose to let go of feelings of worry and fear and replace them with feelings of positivity, optimism, confidence and "can do" about working through any of your life's challenges.

4. View life through the eyes of awe and wonder like a small child. Know beyond a shadow of a doubt that all things are truly possible.

5. Briefly acknowledge what you don't want, and then identify what you prefer instead. Use your innate creativity to chart a path to find ways to manifest these positive preferences.

6. Totally let go things that no longer serve you. Feelings and emotions like fear, worry, resentment, anger, judgment, criticism, guilt, shame and blame have no place in your life. When you release and let go of these emotional burdens, you can replace them with the wonderful qualities of love, joy, acceptance, peace, caring, compassion and happiness.

7. Cultivate patience. Rather than judging people for what they haven't accomplished, support them in the positive attributes that they have now.

8. Love others unconditionally, even when others are less than loving toward you. Over time, this will create positive change within the relationship. I have seen this happen very often when seemingly "hopeless" relationships transform into kind, loving and nurturing friendships and family relationships.

Accentuate the Positive

I'm sure you've heard the expression "do unto others as you would have them do unto you." I think this is a wonderful credo to live by. Unfortunately, in my experience, many women seem to have an easier time with "unto others" than with "unto yourself."

So often I hear women say things about themselves, their bodies, and even their talents, which seem to be self-denigrating. We are constantly criticizing ourselves for not being good enough, smart enough, beautiful enough, or thin enough. My women friends are always jokingly offering to give each other transplants of their most disliked body parts—usually the breasts, behinds, and stomachs. This can create a great deal of depression, low self-esteem and undermine your sense of confidence about yourself if you practice this mindset.

It makes me wonder why this trait is so common among women, and what, if anything, we can do to treat ourselves in a more accepting, caring, and nurturing way. Much of this stems from childhood, when women are often programmed for self-criticism by hearing their own mothers' subtle (or not so subtle) messages of feeling somehow unworthy in their own lives—no matter how accomplished we or our mothers actually are. My own mother, who was a beautiful and accomplished woman and also a medical doctor, did this when I was growing up. This is how deeply negative programming can reach!

Add to this society's impossible standards regarding how a woman should look-- rail-thin, with flawless skin and perfectly coiffed hair—and it should come as no surprise that most women are in a constant self-dialogue of criticism and scorn.

Stop the Negative Self-Talk

When this type of negative self-talk becomes the norm rather than the exception, it can become downright abusive. I'm not referring to physical abuse, but a tendency for a woman to turn emotional violence on herself. Before you wave this off as something that doesn't apply to you, ask yourself these questions:

1. Do you set impossibly high standards for yourself?

2. Do you have higher expectations of yourself than of others?

3. Do you see a friend as "pleasantly plump" but yourself as obese?

4. Do you fixate on a particular aspect of your appearance that most people probably don't even notice?

5. Do you find that if a friend or loved one makes a mistake, or does something hurtful or unwise, you have compassion for her, but if you do something similar, you think of yourself as "stupid" "a loser" or a "failure"?

If you can take an objective look in the mirror and admit that you are harder on yourself than you are on anybody else in your life, then you are at an emotional fork in the road. And there's more at stake than your self-esteem. In fact, the path you choose may determine your level of anxiety and stress and even your physical health.

Research has repeatedly linked our level of self-esteem to emotional and physical well-being. According to a study published in the *Journal of Aging and Health*, positive psychological states and self-image were actually protective against health problems in older adults. Similarly, research from the *Journal of the American Medical Association* found that negative emotions, such as self-criticism, can cause a reduction in blood flow to the heart. And, a study in the *British Journal of Psychiatry* found a higher risk of depression in women with a negative self-image.

Start Loving Yourself

For optimal emotional and physical health and to banish depression, it's important that you send positive messages to your body that reinforce your sense of self-worth and self-love. Try to put to rest any emotional issues you have that are chronic and self-destructive in nature, such as self-criticism and setting yourself up for a lifetime of failures by setting standards that no woman could possibly achieve.

The trouble is most women have tried to live up to unrealistic expectations for so long that the concept of self-deprecation has become deeply ingrained in their minds. As a result, even when you intellectually understand that you need to stop being so hard on yourself, in many cases you find that you simply can't stop. The habit of putting yourself down is so embedded in your mind that the self-destructive thought processes and behaviors have become an involuntary reflex.

My colleague Stacey is a good example. Stacey is a highly accomplished and successful woman. She has an Ivy League doctoral degree, seven published books, hundreds of magazine and scholarly journal articles to her credit, and has been happily married for more than 30 years. She also has a negative and sad secret: She believes she's unworthy and not good enough. She thinks she's the only one who knows, and she works hard to keep it that way. If someone asks her a question, she diligently researches the answer rather than admitting she doesn't know. If she makes a mistake, everything she's ever done right pales in comparison. If someone criticizes her, she can't get it out of her mind.

Contrast Stacey with the mother of one of my college friends. When you were around Rachel, she made you think she was absolutely the most beautiful woman in the world. However, she wasn't particularly attractive in a conventional sense. In fact, some people might have considered her dowdy and plain.

A wise and perceptive woman who was a close friend of the family told me a bit about Rachel's background. She grew up poor, with parents who had very little education. Yet she was an extremely accomplished woman in both her professional and personal life. She had several advanced academic degrees, a high-powered career, and a husband, family, and friends who adored her. Most fascinating to me, however, was the sheer joy she took in herself and everyone around her. It was infectious, and she made us all feel good when we were in her presence.

What's her secret? According to the family friend, despite their own lack of wealth and accomplishment, Rachel's parents had told her from day one how beautiful, capable, and intelligent she was, and that she could achieve anything she wanted. It was a wonderful, positive programming that imprinted Rachel in the deepest way. The good news is that you can create this positive programming, too, no matter what your age or what you perceive are the level of accomplishments in your own life!!

As these two stories show, the key to loving yourself is to reprogram your mind with a new belief system. To do this, you need to redefine your circle of loved ones to include one very special, important, and hard working person—YOU!

Self-Loving Affirmations

I want to share with you a few positive affirmations that reinforce you self-love and self-worth. I use for loving and honoring myself, too. I encourage you to use them to enhance your feelings of self-love and value.

To begin, place your hands in prayer position over your heart. Close your eyes and fill you mind with the most beautiful, peaceful image you can.

Repeat the affirmations five times each. When you feel emotion welling up in your eyes, you'll know that the message got in.

1. I honor and love myself.

2. I am enough.

3. I treat myself with kindness, gentleness, and nurturing.

4. I am worthy.

5. The Divine light of God protects and nurtures me in every way.

6. Every day, I fill myself with feelings of love for God, my friends and family, and all people and creatures on Earth.

7. Kindness and compassion for myself softens and illuminates my heart, casting a warm glow on the world around me.

8. I recognize the light of God in myself, those close to me, and in everyone I encounter on my life journey.

9. I rely on my inner reserves of courage and self-confidence to help make the right choices and decisions.

10. My heart is filled with appreciation and gratitude for all of the blessings that have been bestowed upon me.

The Gift of Giving

Practicing giving to others with a spirit of generosity is a quality that can uplift your spirit and improve your mood. Abundance can manifest many ways, not just financially. You can also feel abundant in your joy, your love and your personal relationships to such an extent that you can pass the overflow on to others.

An act of generosity implies having trust that there is more than enough to go around, as well as confidence in your own inner emotional abundance. It is a great antidote to depression and sadness because it takes our mind off of our own fears and worries and, instead, focuses our attention in a loving way on the needs of others.

Generosity can be physical in which we share our physical belongings with other in need, whether that be money, food, clothing or the gift of our time. It can also be emotional generosity when we make others feel good and worthy, despite feelings that we may sometimes have to the contrary.

I want to share a story of generosity with you that one of my friends and colleagues, David, shared with me. "One night when leaving the hospital with a small group of friends, a woman asked for help in jumping her car battery. After 30 minutes of unsuccessful attempts, I had to leave to attend a prior engagement.

Thankfully, several friends were able to stay on with her. After concluding that her battery was dead, they gave her a ride to her sister's house and then picked up a new car battery with her and drove her back to the hospital where her car was parked. They installed the car battery for her and made sure she was able to get back safely on the road.

After spending several hours helping her, she was completely amazed and touched that strangers would assist her to this extent, without asking for anything in return, no strings attached or preaching. Just "We're glad you are safe and back on the road." I was very touched by their heartfelt generosity when David told me this story

My friend, Jane, is a great example of transforming a negative feeling or reaction into a positive feeling of acceptance for another person and behaving with a spirit of kindness and generosity. Recently, Jane stopped at a local restaurant on her way home from work to pick up dinner for her family. She was feeling guilty about feeding them fast food for the third time that week, but she was running late, her husband was due at a meeting in an hour, and she'd had a particularly hard day.

When she arrived at the counter, the waitress who was supposed to be taking her order was chatting on her cell phone. Jane could tell that the woman had seen her out of the corner of her eye, but she just kept on talking. Finally, after what seemed like an eternity later, she hung up, turned to Jane and said, "What can I get you?" At this point, Jane was so frustrated and angry that she wanted to verbally assault the woman, but she realized that she had a window of opportunity to make a choice: She could fire off a sarcastic comment to mirror her self-righteous anger but she knew that it would unleash a flood of stress hormones into her system.

She realized that her blood pressure was already too high, her stomach was in a knot, and she didn't need her headache to get worse. She also knew that she'd feel bad about losing her temper later on. She decided to reframe her feelings into positive acceptance of the woman in front of her so she took a deep breath, gave her a big, genuine smile and placed her order. Just then her waitress apologized and told Jane that she was on the phone with her family because her mother was ill. Jane expressed her concern for the woman's mother and ended up giving her a big hug. By the time she left with her food, she was feeling much better about herself and the world, in general.

Jane's response ended up being generous to both herself and the woman taking the order. It was generous to be kind and understanding and not to strike out verbally, as she initially felt like doing. It was generous to spare herself the consequences of a flood of stress hormones and remorse. And it was generous to her family not to bring home dinner with a side order of anger and resentment energetically contaminating the food. Instead, she made a positive offering of love.

The Research Tells the Story

Harvard researchers have studied the effects of altruism by taking before-and-after measurements of immune system markers in the saliva of volunteers who watched three films: the first on gardening, the second about war, and the third about Mother Teresa. There was no change in immune markers before or after the first two films, but after the third one, a marker for improved immune function rose dramatically. In other words, just watching someone else be generous is good for your health.

In another landmark study, a researcher from the University of Michigan followed 2,700 people for more than a decade to determine how their social relationships affected their health. He found that more than any other activity, doing volunteer work improved health and increased life expectancy.

Psychologists Allan Luks and Howard Andrews collected surveys from more than 3,000 student volunteers and found that their "helper's high" was followed by a second stage they called the "healthy-helper syndrome." They defined this stage as "a longer-lasting sense of calm and heightened emotional well-being... that is a powerful antidote to anxiety and stress, a key to happiness and optimism, and a way to combat feelings of helplessness and depression."

You Get What You Give

Generosity has a ripple effect—it's contagious. When you give to someone else, they're more likely to give to others. Small acts of generosity, those practiced during your day-to-day life, have a more far-reaching impact than you could ever imagine. When you stop to assist a lone person whose car has broken down and is in obvious distress or help an elderly and unsteady person cross the street, the feel-good endorphins you just created for yourself and someone else will be passed on, possibly to hundreds or even thousands of others. If you could actually follow the ripple effects of your acts of generosity, you would see that they go on forever. In essence, you've just thrown your coin into the cosmic river of life!

10

Stress Reduction for Relief of Chronic Fatigue

In this chapter, I will be sharing with you a number of wonderful and very effective relaxation exercises that will help to repattern your mind and emotions towards more relaxation, peace and joy in your life. If you practice them on a regular basis, they will help to rebuild and restore your energy reserves. You will find that they will help you to deal more effectively with the day-to-days stresses that can put a significant drain on your energy.

Stress is a major trigger for the symptoms of chronic fatigue. If you are already tired because of an imbalance in brain chemistry, hormonal or immune systems imbalances, having too much unmanaged stress in your life can increase your fatigue to a debilitating level. Practicing these nurturing and restorative exercises can help to create more energy reserves within your mind and body and can help to minimize the role of stress in your life, whether minor or more significant.

I have found this to be the case for many of my patients over the years who were suffering from chronic fatigue. The minor everyday stresses that women with normal energy levels handle easily can be overwhelming for a woman whose energy reserves are low. Moreover, significant lifestyle changes — death of a loved one, divorce, job loss, financial problems, major changes in personal relationships — can be very difficult to handle when a woman is chronically fatigued. Practicing effective stress management exercises are very enjoyable to do and will help you better manage and reduce fatigue. Let's take a few minutes and see how stress affects the body.

How Stress Tires the Body

Your reaction to stress is partly determined by how sensitive your autonomic nervous system is. The autonomic nervous system regulates the bodily functions that we are usually unaware of—pulse rate, respiration, muscle tension, glandular function, and circulation of the blood. It is divided into two parts that oppose and complement each other, called the sympathetic and parasympathetic nervous systems.

For example, if fear or excitement speeds up the heart rate too much, the parasympathetic nervous system acts as a control circuit and slows down the heart rate. If the heart slows down too much, then the sympathetic nervous system speeds it up. Thus, the parasympathetic and sympathetic nervous systems have the job of controlling the upper and lower limits of your physiology.

Either major or minor lifestyle upsets may cause an overreaction of the sympathetic system in a woman with chronic fatigue because she has little reserve to deal with such stresses. An easily triggered sympathetic nervous system causes your muscles to tense, your blood vessels to constrict, your adrenal glands to pump out hormones, and your heart and pulse rates to speed up so you can react to an emergency.

If you have an especially stressful life, your sympathetic nervous system may always be poised to react to a crisis. This puts you in a state of constant tension, sometimes known as "fight or flight." In this mode, you tend to react to small stresses the same way you would react to real emergencies. The energy that accumulates in the body to meet this "emergency" must then be discharged to bring your body back into balance.

The end result of the "fight or flight" reaction in women with chronic fatigue is that the repeated process depletes your energy reserves, continuing in a downward spiral that can lead to complete exhaustion. You can break this spiral only by learning to manage stress effectively in a way that protects and even increases your energy level.

Techniques for Relaxation

Many patients have asked me about techniques for coping more effectively with stress. Although I send some women for counseling or psychotherapy, many are looking for practical ways to better manage stress on their own. I have included relaxation and stress reduction exercises in many of my patient programs. The feedback has been very positive. Many of my patients have reported an increased sense of well-being from these self-care techniques. When practiced on a regular basis, they can also help to improve your general health and well-being.

In this chapter, I have included a number of different stress reduction exercises to help relax and quiet your mind and thereby help to restore your energy. I recommend that you try the exercises that most appeal to you and then practice the ones that you enjoy the most on a regular basis.

Handling Negative Thoughts and Feelings

Throughout the day your conscious mind may be barraged with thoughts, feelings, and fantasies about your daily life. Many of these thoughts replay unresolved issues of health, finances, or personal relationships that are causing you anxiety and discomfort. A woman with chronic fatigue can find this relentless mental replay of unresolved issues exhausting. It is important to know how to shut off the constant inner dialogue and quiet the mind.

The first two exercises require you to sit quietly and engage in a simple repetitive activity. By emptying your mind, you give yourself a rest. Meditation allows you to create a state of deep relaxation, which is very healing to the entire body. If you practice these exercises regularly, they can help relieve chronic fatigue by resting your mind and turning off any upsetting thoughts.

The third meditation will help you release tension and relax. If you want to enjoy deep restful sleep, this peaceful meditation will help you relax and unwind. I've seen it create great benefits for both adults and children, alike. It is a very simple, yet effective, exercise

Exercise 1: Concentration

Select an object that you like. It can be a flower or a small piece of your jewelry. Focus all your attention on this object as you inhale and exhale slowly and deeply for one to two minutes. While you are doing this exercise, don't let any other thoughts or feelings enter your mind. At the end of this exercise you will probably feel more peaceful and calmer. Any tension or nervousness that you were feeling upon starting the exercise should be diminished.

Exercise 2: Meditation on Love and Joy

- Sit or lie in a comfortable position. Allow your arms to rest by your sides. Begin to inhale and exhale slowly and deeply with your eyes closed.
- As you inhale, say the word "love" to yourself, and as you exhale, say the word "joy." Draw out the pronunciation of the word so that it lasts for the entire breath: l-l-l-o-o-o-o-v-v-v-e-e-e, j-j-j-o-o-o-y-y-y. Repeating these words as you breathe will help you to concentrate.
- Focus all your attention on your breathing. Notice your chest and abdomen moving in and out.
- If your attention wanders, refocus on your breathing and word repetition.

Continue doing this meditation until you feel very peaceful and relaxed.

Exercise 3: Meditation for Sleep and Relaxation

To begin the meditation, breathe in and out, slowly and deeply. Let the cares of the day fall away.

Now visualize being in your favorite peaceful place, whether it is a garden, meadow, seashore or favorite getaway. Look around you and enjoy the sense of calm and relaxation that you get from being in this beautiful place. You can stay in this place of peace as long as you want.

As you continue to breathe in and out slowly and deeply, let yourself gently fall into a peaceful sleep.

Technique

When women are feeling tired and overwhelmed from too much tension and stress, they often lose a sense of being grounded, literally rooted to the earth. Some women report a sensation of numbness in their legs and feet. They may say that they feel as if they have no legs at all. Perhaps you have experienced these sensations, too, during times of stress.

When you become physically ungrounded by symptoms of emotional distress, it is also very difficult to function mentally. You can have a hard time focusing and concentrating. There is a pervasive sense of "things falling apart." You may even have difficulty working through your projects for the day in an organized manner. It often takes a concentrated effort just to get through the day, accomplishing such basic daily tasks as cooking, house cleaning, taking care of children, or getting to work or school.

This next exercise will help you to ground and focus both physically and mentally. Practicing this exercises will allow you to organize your energies and proceed more effectively with your daily routine during times when you feel more anxious and scattered. You should feel much more stable and focused by the end of this exercise.

Exercise 4: Grounding

Sit upright in a chair. Be sure you are in a comfortable position. Keep your feet slightly apart. Breathe in and out through your nose.

- Inhale deeply. As you breathe in, allow your stomach to relax so that the air flows into your abdomen. Let your stomach balloon out as you breathe in. Visualize the lowest parts of your lungs filling up with air. Hold your inhalation.

- Visualize a golden cord with a golden ball at the end of it running from the base of your spine. Let this golden cord gently and slowly move downwards through the earth, grounding you. You can let it move down as far as you would like, even all the way to the center of the earth.

- Follow the cord and its golden ball in your mind all the way down and see it fasten securely to the earth's center. You can run two golden cords from the bottoms of your feet down to the center of the earth, also, if you would like.

- As you exhale, become aware of your hips, thighs, calves, ankles, and feet. Feel their strength and solidity.

- Repeat this exercise several times until you feel fully present and grounded.

Releasing Muscle Tension

The next three exercises will help you focus on areas in your body that are holding chronic muscle tension and so that you can begin to release it. Often, habitual emotional patterns cause certain muscle groups to tense and tighten. For example, if you have difficulty in expressing feelings or speaking your truth, the neck muscles may become chronically tense. If you are dealing with a lot of fear and worry or repressed anger, you may have episodes of chest pain and tight chest muscles during times when you are feeling upset and are having difficulty expressing it or even handling the situation that is causing these symptoms.

When blocked feelings and emotions cause your muscles to tighten and contract, this limits the movement and flow of energy in the body. Tight muscles have decreased blood circulation and oxygenation and accumulate an excess of waste products, such as carbon dioxide and lactic acid. As a result, muscle tension can be a significant cause of the fatigue that often accompanies chronic stress. The following exercises will help release tension and the blocked emotions held in tight muscles.

Exercise 5: Discovering Muscle Tension

- Lie on your back in a comfortable position. Allow your arms to rest at your sides, palms down, on the surface next to you.

- Raise just the right hand and arm and hold it elevated for 15 seconds.

- Notice if your forearm feels tight and tense or if the muscles are soft and pliable.

- Let your hand and arm drop down and relax. The arm muscles will relax too.

- As you lie still, notice any other parts of your body that feel tense, muscles that feel tight and sore. You may notice a constant dull aching in certain muscles.

Exercise 6: Progressive Muscle Relaxation

- Lie on your back in a comfortable position. Allow your arms to rest at your sides, palms down, on the surface next to you.

- Inhale and exhale slowly and deeply.

- Clench your hands into fists and hold them for a few seconds.

- Then let your hands relax. On relaxing, see a golden light flowing into the entire body, making all your muscles soft and pliable.

- Now, tense and relax the following parts of your body in this order: face, shoulders, back, stomach, pelvis, legs, feet, and toes. Hold each part tensed for a few seconds and then relax your body for 15 seconds before going on to the next part.

- Finish the exercise by shaking your hands and imagining the remaining tension flowing out of your fingertips.

Exercise 7: Release of Muscle Tension and Stress

Lie in a comfortable position. Allow your arms to rest at your sides, palms down. Inhale and exhale slowly and deeply with your eyes closed.

- Become aware of your feet, ankles, and legs. Notice if these parts of your body have any muscle tension or tightness. If so, how does the tense part of your body feel? Is it viselike, knotted, cold or numb? Do you notice any feelings, such as hurt, upset, fear or anger coming up or even just a feeling of tension as you focus on that part of your body? Breathe into that part of your body until you feel it relax. Release any feelings or emotions with your breathing, continuing until they begin to decrease in intensity and fade.

- Next, move your awareness to your hips, pelvis, and lower back. Notice any tension or anxious feelings located in that part of your body. Breathe into your hips and pelvis until you feel them relax. Release any negative emotions as you breathe in and out. You should begin to feel more peace and calm as you continue to breathe deeply and slowly, in and out.

- Focus on your abdomen and chest. Notice any tense or upset feelings located in this area and let them drop away as you breathe in and out. Continue to release any upsetting feelings located in your abdomen or chest.

- Finally, focus on your head, neck, arms, and hands. Note any tension in this area and release it. With your breathing, release any negative feelings blocked in this area until you can't feel them anymore. Let them be replaced by feelings of peace, calm and relaxation.

- When you have finished releasing tension throughout the body, continue deep breathing and relaxing for another minute or two. At the end of this exercise, you should feel lighter and more energized.

Erasing Stress and Tension

Often the situations and beliefs that make us feel anxious, fearful and tense feel large and insurmountable. We tend to form pictures in our mind that empower stress. In these images, we look tiny and helpless, while the stressors look huge and unsolvable. This can drain your energy and add to your feelings of tiredness and fatigue.

You can change these mental images and cut stressors down to size. The next two exercises will help you to gain mastery over stress by learning to shrink it or even erase it with your mind. This places stress in a much more manageable and realistic perspective and allows you to focus on creative solutions to your issues and challenges. These two exercises will help engender a sense of power and mastery, thereby reducing worry and anxiety and restoring a sense of calm.

Exercise 8: Shrinking Stress

- Sit or lie in a comfortable position. Breathe slowly and deeply. Visualize a situation, person, or even a belief that makes you feel anxious and tense.

- As you do this, you might see a person's face, a place you're afraid to go, or simply a dark cloud. Where do you see this stressful picture? Is it above you, to one side, or in front of you? How does it look? Is it big or little, dark or light? Does it have certain colors?

- Now slowly begin to shrink the stressful picture. Continue to see the stressful picture shrinking until it is so small that it can literally be held in the palm of your hand. Hold your hand out in front of you, and place the picture in the palm of your hand.

- If the stressor has a characteristic sound, hear it getting tiny and soft. As it continues to shrink, its voice or sounds become almost inaudible.

- Now the stressful picture is so small it can fit on your finger. Watch it shrink from there until it finally turns into a little dot and disappears.

- Often this exercise causes feelings of amusement, as well as relaxation, as the feared stressor shrinks, gets less intimidating, and finally disappears.

- Then visualize every cell of your body being filled with a golden light. This golden light is Divine love and protection. Know that you are loved and are always being watched over and protected. When you shrink the stressors in your life, you can more easily feel and become aware of God's love for you. Continue to breathe in this Divine golden light until you feel peaceful and calm.

Exercise 9: Erasing Stress

- Sit or lie in a comfortable position. Breathe slowly and deeply.

- Visualize a situation, a person, or even a belief (such as, "I'm afraid to go to the shopping mall" or "I'm scared to mix with other people at parties") that causes you to feel anxious and fearful.

- As you do this you might see a specific person, an actual place, or simply shapes and colors. Where do you see this stressful picture? Is it below you, to the side, in front of you? How does it look? Is it big or little, dark or light, or does it have a specific color?

- Imagine that a large eraser, like the kind used to erase chalk marks, has just floated into your hand. Actually feel and see the eraser in your hand. Take the eraser and begin to rub it over the area where the stressful picture is located. As the eraser rubs out the stressful picture it fades, shrinks, and finally disappears. When you can no longer see the stressful picture, simply continue to focus on your deep breathing for another minute, inhaling and exhaling slowly and deeply.

- Then, see yourself handling the situation or person who formerly caused you distress with self-confidence and mastery. Know that you are empowered and capable of handling any situation that you choose and that you can create positive solutions to every perceived issue or challenge.

- Let feelings of peace and calm fill your mind as you continue to breathe slowly and deeply.

Healing the Inner Child

Many of our fears, worries and anxieties come from our inner child rather than our adult self. Sometimes it is difficult to realize that the emotional upsets that can cause so much suffering are actually feelings that are left over or originate from childhood fears, traumas, and experiences. When unhealed, they remain with us into adulthood, causing emotional distress over issues that competent "grown-up" people feel they should be able to handle. These unresolved issues drain our energy and can contribute greatly to chronic fatigue and tiredness.

For example, fear of the dark, fear of being unlovable, and fear of rejection often originate in early dysfunctional or unhappy experiences with our parents, siblings or other relationships. They can also arise from difficult life circumstances such as family poverty or lack that we experienced when we were young.

While these deep, unresolved emotional issues may sometimes require counseling, particularly if they are causing extreme anxiety and stress episodes, there is much that we can do for ourselves to heal childhood wounds. The next exercise helps you to get in touch with your own inner child and facilitates the healing process.

Exercise 10: Healing the Inner Child

- Sit or lie in a comfortable position. Breathe slowly and deeply. Begin to get in touch with where your inner child resides. Is she located in your abdomen, in your chest, or by your side? (This may actually be the part of your body where you feel the most fear and anxiety) How old is she? Can you see what clothes she is wearing? What are her emotions? Is she upset, anxious, sad, or angry? Is she withdrawn and quiet?

- Now visualize holding her in your arms or putting her on your lap. See yourself cuddling her and treating her with love and tenderness. Maybe she would like a toy animal or a doll that you can give to her. If she is sad or upset, let her know how special and precious she is to you and how much you love her. Continue to hold her and cuddle or rock her in your arms until you feel her becoming more peaceful and calm.

- Then begin to fill your inner child with a peaceful, healing, golden light. Let this beautiful, loving light fills every cell in her body. Watch her body relax.

- As you leave your inner child feeling peaceful, return your focus to your breathing. Spend a minute inhaling and exhaling deeply and slowly. If you like working with your inner child, return to visit her often!

Visualization

The next five exercises use visualization as a therapeutic method to help restore the physical and mental health of your body and mind. The first two focus on using color. Color therapy has a long history of being used to promote healing. In many fascinating studies, scientists have exposed subjects to specific colors, either directly through exposure to light therapy, or through changing the color of their environment.

Research done throughout the world has shown that color therapy can have a profoundly positive effect on health, well-being and even affect your mood. It can stimulate the endocrine glands, the immune system, nervous system and help to balance your emotions and mood. Visualizing color in a specific part of the body can also have a powerful therapeutic effect, too, and can be a good stress management technique for relief of chronic fatigue and restoring energy.

The first exercise uses the color blue, which provides a calming and relaxing effect. For women with chronic fatigue who are carrying a lot of physical and emotional tension, blue helps to diminish the "fight or flight" response. (This response stresses the adrenal glands and, over time, leads to exhaustion.) Blue also calms physiological functions such as pulse rate, breathing, and perspiration, and relaxes the mood. It should be used primarily by fatigued women who are chronically tense, anxious, irritable, or carry a lot of muscle tension.

The second exercise uses the color red, which can benefit all women who have fatigue. Red stimulates all the endocrine glands, including the pituitary and adrenal glands. It heightens senses such as smell and taste. Autonomic nervous system function speeds up with increased blood flow and blood pressure; metabolic rate increases, too. Emotionally, red is linked to vitality and high-energy states. I often do the red visualization when I am tired and need a pick-me-up.

The third exercise helps you to use the power of visualization to restore your health and energy. When you visualize your body as healthy, strong, and vital, you begin to lay down the mental blueprint for better health.

This technique of actually imaging your body the way that you want it to be has been used in the treatment of cancer as well as other serious diseases. This technique was pioneered by Carl Simonton, M.D., a cancer radiation therapist. A number of his patients, after using this technique to stimulate their immune systems and shrink their tumors, saw their diseases go into remission. In this exercise you use the same type of visualization to relieve chronic fatigue.

The last two exercises use positive visualization to engender feelings of love and connection to God, the Divine Source of love, peace, joy and compassion. These two exercises use the incredible power of visualization to help eliminate feelings of chronic stress, depression and overwhelm, and replace them with positive, nurturing and life enhancing emotions.

The visualization on love will greatly enhance your mood and assist you in eliminating unwanted emotions like fear, stress and anxiety by helping you to nurture and lovingly care for yourself. The visualization on Divine healing water was created to reinforce your connection to God, our Creator.

These are two of my favorite exercises for their great benefits of elevating our thoughts and feelings in a positive way. I always feel loving, peaceful and calm when I do them myself.

Exercise 11: Tension Release Through Color

- Sit or lie in a comfortable position, your arms resting at your sides. As you take a deep breath, visualize that the earth below you is filled with the color blue. Now imagine that you are opening up energy centers on the bottom of your feet. As you inhale, visualize the soft blue color filling up your feet. When your feet are completely filled with the color blue, then bring the color up through your ankles, legs, pelvis, and lower back.

- Each time you exhale, see the blue color leaving through your lungs, carrying any tension and stress with it. See the tension dissolve into the air.

- Continue to inhale blue into your abdomen, chest, shoulders, arms, neck, and head. Exhale the blue slowly out of your lungs. Repeat this entire process five times and then relax for a few minutes.

Exercise 12: Energizing Through Color

- Sit or lie in a comfortable position, your arms resting easily at your sides. As you take a deep breath, visualize a big balloon above your head filled with a bright red healing energy. Imagine that you pop this balloon so all the bright red energy is released.

- As you inhale, see the bright red color filling up your head. It fills up your brain, your face, and the bones of your skull. Let the bright red color pour in until your head is ready to overflow with color. Then let the red color flow into your neck, shoulders, arms, and chest. As you exhale, breathe the red color out of your lungs, taking any tiredness and fatigue with it. Breathe any feeling of fatigue out of your body.

- As you inhale, continue to bring the bright, energizing red color into your abdomen, pelvis, lower back, legs, and feet until your whole body is filled with red. Exhale the red color out of your lungs, continuing to release any feeling of fatigue. Repeat this process five times. At the end of this exercise, you should feel more energized and vibrant. Your mental energy should feel more vitalized and clear.

Exercise 13: Visualization for a Healthy Body

When you visualize your body as healthy, strong, and vital, you begin to lay down the mental blueprint for better health. This technique of actually imaging your body the way that you want it to be has been used in the treatment of cancer as well as other serious diseases.

- Close your eyes and begin to breathe deeply, slowly inhaling and exhaling. Feel your body begin to relax.

- Imagine that you are looking in a mirror. Actually see yourself in your mind's eye.

- Visualize your face radiant and full of vibrant energy. Your skin is glowing and healthy looking. Your eyes are bright and clear. Your face is confident and smiling. You feel tension-free and in command of yourself.

- As you see yourself in the mirror, you are pleased with how vibrant and energized you look. You feel you could handle any problems that come along with ease.

- Now, visualize your entire body and see a current of energy running through every part of your body. See yourself radiating health and well-being. Look at your breasts, abdomen, hips, legs, and feet. Visualize the energy and vitality running through your entire body. Your body looks strong, sturdy, and healthy. You feel optimistic and confident. Your mood is calm and relaxed.

- Now, return your focus again on breathing deeply, in and out. After 15 or 20 seconds, open your eyes and continue to relax for a minute or two.

Exercise 13: Loving Yourself

- To do this visualization, find a quiet spot where you can sit or lie comfortably. As you take a deep breath, focus on the area of your heart (located just to the left of the center of your chest).

- As you inhale and exhale slowly and deeply, close your eyes and envision your heart as a luminous, emerald-green jewel glowing with love and sending out brilliant light from behind your breastbone, where your heart resides.

- As you breathe slowly, begin to fill your heart with love. Feel the area surrounding your heart soften and expand as you fill it with loving and peaceful energy.

- Next, send love and appreciation to every part of your body, even the parts that you are concerned about or feel are less than lovable. They are all parts or you and worthy of the deepest love and caring.

- Breathe love and appreciation into your head, neck, shoulders, chest and down your arms and hands. Send this loving and healing breathe next into your abdomen, hips, legs and feet.

- Continue loving and appreciating yourself until you feel your entire body overflowing with love.

- Now gently open your eyes and slowly begin to move around again. Enjoy the feelings of love, peace and gratitude you have created.

Exercise 14: Divine Healing Water

- Sit or lie in a comfortable position, with your arms resting gently by your sides.

- Now, close your eyes and breathe deeply. Let your breathing be slow and relaxed.

- Visualize a river of living water flowing gently through you. This is Divine healing water, full of God's light and love.

  Feel this healing water flow into every cell of your body, cleansing you of all cares and worries, bringing you the deepest peace.

- Let this healing water flow through your head, renewing your mind and then moving into your neck and shoulders. As it moves through you, it carries away any tension and tightness.

- Then feel this Divine water flow gently into your chest and down your arms and hands, and then into your abdomen, bringing with it healing and life energy.

- Next, let this water move into your hips and pelvis and down into your legs and feet.

- As this Divine water leaves your body, all darkness is disappearing and is being replaced by light, love and happiness.

- Let this Divine healing water flow through you as long as you would like it to. Continue this process until you feel totally at peace and deeply relaxed.

- • Let this Divine healing water flow through you as long as you would like it to. Continue this process until you feel totally at peace and deeply relaxed.

Affirmations

The following two exercises give you healthful affirmations that can be very useful for women with chronic fatigue. When I work with a patient, I always stress the important connection between the mind and body. Your state of health is determined in part by the thousands of mental messages you send yourself each day with your thoughts. To truly heal from any health problem, the mind and body must work together in a positive way. It is not enough to follow a good diet and take the medication that a physician prescribes. When your body believes it is sick, it behaves as if it is sick.

For example, if you have a peptic ulcer and your belief is that you can never really get well, the ulcer pain will worsen. If you believe that your arthritis symptoms can only increase in severity, your joints will continue to be stiff and uncomfortable. Similarly, if you are constantly criticizing the way you look, your lack of self-love will be reflected in your body. Your shoulders will slump and your countenance will be lackluster.

Affirmations provide a method to change these negative belief systems to thoughts that reinforce the positives in your life. They uplift your thinking to appreciation and gratitude for all that you have in your life and to see yourself for the special and wonderful woman that you are. The positive statements contained in affirmations replace the anxiety and stress inducing messages that can exhaust you. Instead, fill your mind with thoughts that make you feel good about yourself and your life.

The first affirmation exercise gives you a series of statements to promote a sense of physical health and well-being. Using these affirmations may create a feeling of greater vigor and vitality by changing your negative beliefs about your body and health into positive ones. The second affirmation exercise helps to promote self-esteem and self-confidence. This is important in healing a low energy level and depressed mood. Many women with chronic fatigue lose their self-confidence and feel depressed and defeated by their condition. They feel frustrated and somehow at fault for not finding a solution. You can use either or both exercises on a regular basis to promote positive, energy enhancing thoughts.

Exercise 16: Energizing Body Affirmations

- My body is strong and healthy.

- My thoughts and feelings are positive and life affirming.

- My mood is calm and relaxed.

- I wake up each day grateful for all the wonderful things that God has given me.

- I can create positive solutions to every issue in my life.

- I have all the energy that I need. My body is constantly renewing itself with vibrant energy.

- My brain chemistry is healthy and balanced and supports my mood in a positive and joyful manner.

- My endocrine glands are healthy and strong. They function perfectly and make just the right amount of hormones that I need to be radiantly healthy.

- My thyroid gland, ovaries and adrenals are becoming stronger and healthier each day. My glands are all working together to create health and balance in my body and mind.

- My body chemistry is balanced and healthy.

- My immune system functions perfectly and protects me from infections and allergies.

- I handle stress and tension appropriately and effectively.

- I eat a well-balanced and nutritious diet.

- I enjoy eating delicious and healthful food.

- I do regular exercise in a relaxed and enjoyable manner.

Exercise 17: Self-Esteem Affirmations

- I am filled with energy, vitality, and self-confidence.

- I am pleased with how I handle my health needs.

- I know exactly how to manage my daily schedule to accommodate my energy level.

- I listen to my body's needs and regulate my activity level to take care of my body's needs.

- I love and honor my body

- I fill my mind with positive and self-nourishing thoughts.

- I am a wonderful and worthy person.

- I deserve health and vitality

- I have total confidence in my ability to heal myself.

- I feel radiant with abundant energy and vitality.

- The world around me is full of radiant beauty and abundance.

- I am attracted people and situations that support and nurture me.

- I appreciate the positive people and situations that are currently in my life.

- I love and honor myself.

- I enjoy my abundant energy and vitality.

Putting Your Stress-Reduction Program Together

This chapter has introduced you to many different ways to support and nourish your mind and body to combat chronic fatigue. You can try each exercise or do the ones that appeal to you the most. You will find the combination that works best for you. Over time, they will help to relieve fatigue inducing stress and tension and repattern your emotional responses. These exercises will help to eliminate negative feelings and beliefs while changing them into positive, self-nurturing new ones. Your feelings of fatigue and tiredness should diminish and your ability to cope with stress will improve tremendously with regular practice.

11

Breathing Exercises

Therapeutic breathing is of major benefit to women suffering from chronic fatigue. In fact, I strongly recommend its use in any chronic fatigue healing program. Women who are tired tend to restrict their movements in general. They exercise less, go out socially less frequently, and even restrict their household tasks. They spend more time lying on the bed or couch.

When movement is limited in this way, breathing tends to become shallow and restricted. Instead of the deep abdominal breathing that we see with healthy aerobic activity, fatigued women may find that they practically stop breathing altogether and hold their breath for prolonged periods of time without even realizing it. The end result is a decrease in oxygen levels in the body, poorer blood circulation, muscle tension and a decrease in metabolic activity of the cells. This can worsen chronic fatigue and tiredness.

Deep, slow abdominal breathing is essential for taking in large amounts of oxygen from the environment. Oxygen moves from the air you inhale, first into your lungs, and then into your circulation, where it binds to the red blood cells while traveling through the arteries and veins. Oxygen enables the cells to produce and utilize energy as well as remove waste products through the production of carbon dioxide, which you eliminate by exhaling. Your entire body needs optimal levels of oxygen for its normal cycle of building, repair, and elimination.

Therapeutic breathing exercises help enhance oxygenation and healthy metabolic function, thereby improving energy. I recommend that you try the exercises that most appeal to you in this chapter, then practice on a regular basis the ones you find that you enjoy the most. Pay attention to your breathing habits. If you catch yourself breathing shallowly or infrequently, correct this tendency by using the breathing techniques in this chapter. It is important to do the breathing exercises in a slow and regular manner. Find a comfortable position before beginning the exercises. Unless otherwise directed, keep your arms and legs uncrossed and your back straight.

Exercise 1: Deep Abdominal Breathing

Abdominal breathing is a very important technique for the relief of chronic fatigue and for improving energy and vitality. Deep, slow breathing brings adequate oxygen, the fuel for metabolic activity, to all the tissues of your body. In contrast, rapid, shallow breathing decreases the oxygen supply and keeps you tired and devitalized. Deep breathing helps release tension and anxiety and relaxes the entire body. It also helps balance many other physiological processes such as pulse rate and hormonal output so that you can conserve and build your energy level, thereby healing chronic fatigue.

- Lie flat on your back with your knees pulled up. Keep your feet slightly apart. Try to breathe in and out through your nose.

- Inhale deeply. As you breathe in, allow your stomach to relax so that the air flows into your abdomen. Your stomach should balloon out as you breathe in. Visualize your lungs filling up with air so that your chest swells out.

- Imagine that the air you breathe is filling your body with energy.

- Exhale deeply. As you breathe out, let your stomach and chest collapse. Imagine the air being pushed out, first from your abdomen and then from your lungs.

- Repeat this exercise 10 times.

Exercise 2: Energy Breathing

This exercise combines imagery with deep breathing. As you visualize the energizing effects that breathing has on your body, you actually begin to lay down a mental blueprint for enhanced health and well-being. This exercise should leave you feeling peaceful with a greater degree of energy.

- Sit upright in a chair or lie flat on your back with your knees pulled up. Keep your feet slightly apart. Breathe in and out through your nose, if possible.

- Inhale deeply. As you breathe in, allow your stomach to relax so that the air flows into your abdomen. Let your stomach balloon out as you breathe in. Visualize the lowest parts of your lungs filling up with air.

- Imagine that the air you are breathing is filled with energy and vitality. Visualize this energy as a golden color Feel the vitality filling every cell of your body. It fills you with a sensation of warmth and healing. See the golden energy healing your body.

- Now, exhale deeply. As you breathe out, imagine the air being pushed out from the bottom of your lungs to the top.

- Repeat this sequence until your entire body feels relaxed and your breathing is slow and regular.

Exercise 3: Hara Breathing

In the traditional Chinese healing method, the hara is one of the most important centers of vitality. In fact, it is called the "Sea of Energy." The hara point, located three finger-widths below the naval, is considered the center of the body. Stimulation of the hara point helps to strengthen the body, as well as improve energy and endurance. Hara breathing nourishes and energizes the internal organs, improving health in general as well as decreasing chronic fatigue and tiredness.

- Sit upright in a chair, your arms at your sides. First, find the hara point with your fingers. Then, as you inhale deeply, draw breath into your lower abdomen and focus on concentrating your breath into the hara point. Feel the hara point expand and energize.

- As you exhale, release the energy from the hara point so that it moves from your lower abdomen and then circulates throughout your body.

- Repeat this exercise for several minutes—drawing breath and energy into the hara point as you inhale, then circulating energy throughout your body as you exhale.

Exercise 4: Breath of Fire

This short, rapid breathing technique is used in stretches to charge the body with immediate energy. This exercise also energizes the nervous system and stimulates blood circulation. Only do this exercise if you feel comfortable doing it since it is done rapidly.

- Sit upright in a chair, your arms at your sides, palms up. As you inhale, fill your abdomen with a deep breath. Then breathe rapidly out through your nose, exhaling one short breath every second or two. As you breathe out, contract your abdomen by pumping in and out until your lungs are empty.

- Repeat several times until you feel energized and fully awake and present.

Exercise 5: Complete Body Breathing

This exercise promotes energy and vitality by directing your breath into every part of your body. This helps release stress and muscle tension in parts of your body that you are not even aware are tense which help to increase the energy of the entire body. Doing this exercise reinforces the importance of the body functioning as a whole, integrated unit for optimal health and well-being. It also expands the electromagnetic field of the body through the use of color.

- Sit or lie in a comfortable position. Now, take a deep breath and imagine that you are opening up energy centers on the bottoms of your feet.

- As you inhale, visualize a bright red colored energy filling up your feet. Draw this color up your legs and into your pelvic area and your lower back. As you exhale through your lungs, see this color flow out of your body and fill the air around you. Release any feeling of tiredness, depression or negative feelings or or emotions as you exhale. Continue doing this until the lower part of your body feeling clear and bright.

- Now inhale the bright red color up into your abdomen, chest, shoulders, and arms. See it filling your neck and head. As you exhale, see the bright red color flow out through your lungs and fill the air around you. As you breathe out, release any tiredness or negative thoughts and feelings until you feel bright and energized.

- You can repeat this process several times.

Exercise 6: Glandular Breathing

Chronic fatigue often depletes endocrine gland function. Women with depleted endocrine glands may not only feel tired, but may also be prone to hormone imbalances and infections, because the endocrine glands help to regulate healthy female hormonal health and immunity. Optimal endocrine function is very important for disease resistance, vitality, and energy.

This exercise helps stimulate and energize your endocrine glands through the use of color breathing. When you direct your breath into the endocrine glands and visualize them being stimulated by the color, the glands receive better oxygenation and blood circulation. Nutrient flow to the glands is improved, as is the removal of waste products and toxins. The use of color increases the glands' health and energy.

- Sit upright in a chair, your arms at your sides, palms up. Imagine that there is a large red cloud above your head. This is a bright, vibrant tone of red that sparkles with energy. As you inhale deeply, see the color red from this cloud flowing into your head and concentrating in the hypothalamus. The hypothalamus is the master endocrine gland of the body that regulates the function of all the other glands. It is located in the area between the eyes, deep in the middle of the brain

- As the hypothalamus begins to overflow with color, exhale and breathe the red out of your lungs, filling the air around you.

- As you inhale again, breathe the bright red color into your pituitary, an important endocrine gland located in your brain, right below the hypothalamus. Fill the pituitary with this color until it overflows. Then exhale deeply

- As you continue to inhale the bright red color, let it flow into your thyroid gland, located in your neck, then into your thymus gland, located in the middle of your chest.

- Finally, let the color energize your adrenal glands, located in the middle of your back above the kidneys, and then your ovaries, located in the pelvis.

- When you finish this exercise, relax for a few minutes.

Exercise 7: Emotional Healing Breath

I have seen, during my years of medical practice, that emotional stress is a significant trigger for chronic fatigue. This exercise uses breathing to help you release negative feelings such as chronic anger, hurt, or other upsets you may be harboring. The more time you spend cleansing old negative emotional patterns, the less impact these feelings will have on your energy levels.

- Lie flat on your back with your knees pulled up. Keep your feet slightly apart. Try to breathe in and out through your nose.

- Inhale deeply and see yourself enveloped in a soft white light. Breathe this light into every cell of your body. This is a cleansing light and can help wash away fear, anger, anxiety, and other negative feelings.

- As you exhale deeply, feel the light washing these emotions away

- Repeat this exercise until you feel emotionally peaceful and clear.

Exercise 8: Muscle Tension Release Breathing

I want to share with you a wonderful exercise that will help you to get in touch with and release any muscle tension and tightness and bring your body back into a state of healthy balance. Often when you are anxious and upset, you may unconsciously tense up muscles throughout the entire body. The neck, shoulders, lower back, hips and other areas of the body are particularly vulnerable.

Muscle tension often occurs in response to the stresses of the day or from sitting in one position for hours at the desk or computer and even after doing vigorous exercise. After doing this meditation, you will feel more peaceful and relaxed!

- Sit or lie in a comfortable position. Allow your arms to rest at your sides, palms down and inhale and exhale slowly and deeply.

- Become aware of your feet, ankles, and legs. Notice if these parts of your body have any muscle tension or tightness. Breathe into that part of your body until you feel it relax.

- Next, move your awareness into your hips, pelvis, and lower back. Note any tension there. Breathe into your hips and pelvis until you feel them relax. Release any emotional stress as you breathe in and out.

- Focus on your abdomen and chest. Notice any tension or tightness located in this area and let it drop away as you breathe in and out. Continue to breathe into this area until your chest and abdomen feel relaxed.

- Finally, focus on your head, neck, arms, and hands. Note any tension in this area and release it. With your breathing, release any negative emotions blocked in this area until you feel peaceful and calm.

- When you have finished releasing tension throughout the body, continue deep breathing and relaxing for another minute or two. At the end of this exercise, you should feel lighter, relaxed and more energized.

Exercise 9: Divine Healing Breath

This is one of my favorite and most inspirational breathing and meditation exercises. I always feel uplifted when I do this exercise. It is a beautiful meditation on filling yourself with the Divine light and love of God. This meditation will also help you release any tension or negativity from your mind and fill you with wonderful feelings of peace and joy.

- Begin the meditation by finding a quiet place. It can be a peaceful room in your house or office or even a beautiful spot in your backyard. Then, sit or lie in a comfortable position, with your arms resting gently by your sides.

- Close your eyes and breathe deeply. Let your breathing be slow and relaxed. Visualize yourself as a flower in the sun, opening yourself to God's light and love. Feel this Divine light surrounding you and enfolding you, filling every cell of your body with love.

- As this light fills and nurtures you, you are being cleansed of all cares and worries. This Divine light is dispelling all darkness as it gently and lovingly restores you to a state of health, balance and peace.

- Visualize this Divine light, bringing brightness and clarity into your mind, your head and then your neck and shoulders. As it moves through you, it carries away any tension and tightness.

- As you continue to breathe deeply and slowly, feel the warmth of this light as it moves into your chest and down your arms and hands, and then into your abdomen, bringing with it healing and protection.

- Next, let this Divine light move into your hips and pelvis and finally down into your legs and feet.

- Let this Divine light move through you as long as you would like it to. Continue this process until you feel totally at peace and deeply relaxed.

- Know that God is always with you, caring for you and loving you always.

Exercise 10: Depression Release Breathing

Depression often accompanies chronic fatigue. When a woman is tired, often her mood is low, too. It is hard to feel enthusiastic and high-spirited about life when you have no energy and vitality supporting your mental processes. This next exercise helps to elevate your mood and enhance emotional well-being through focused breathing.

- Sit upright in a chair. Your arms are crossed in front of your chest with your fingers touching the upper outer area of your chest. Your wrist crosses over your heart chakra, which is the energy center for emotions and feelings in traditional Chinese healing models.

- As you inhale, imagine a golden light filling your heart center with a warm, loving feeling. As you exhale, breathe out depression and low spirits.

- As you inhale again, draw this golden light up through your neck and into your head. See it illuminating your head with a soft, peaceful glow. Feel any depression or negative thoughts dissolving as the golden light fills every cell in your brain.

- As you exhale, breathe the golden light out through the top of your head and see it form a shimmering cloud of energy around your entire body.

- Repeat the exercise 5 times.

Putting Your Breathing Exercise Program Together

In this chapter, I have shared with you many wonderful and enjoyable breathing exercises to help reduce chronic fatigue and tiredness as well as support improved health and more peace and joy. You may want to try each exercise once or choose those that most appeal to you. I recommend practicing breathing exercises on a regular basis for their great anxiety and stress reducing benefits. These exercises can help you even if you practice them only a few minutes each day. Over time, healthy breathing habits will become automatic and will also greatly benefit your general health.

12

Light Therapy for Chronic Fatigue

One of the most powerful ways to relieve fatigue, lack of energy, pain and depression is to use red light therapy devices. I love this type of therapy because it is so gentle, yet very effective in helping to bring women back into healthy balance, especially when used in conjunction with my anti-fatigue diet, nutritional supplement program and other self-care treatments that I discuss in this book.

I first became aware of the existence of colored light therapy as a third year medical student. At that time, I was doing my pediatric rotation, and I learned that colored light, specifically blue light therapy, was being used to treat jaundice in premature infants in order to protect them from brain damage.

The idea that such a gentle and non-invasive therapy could help save the lives of newborns was very intriguing to me. I decided to delve into the research and discover what other health conditions this amazing therapy could treat. I began to intensively study the medical research on colored light, along with a very good friend of mine who was a biophysicist at NASA and had a similar interest in this area. We obtained a red light laser and he and I performed research studies on plant growth and laser therapy. My interest in the healing benefits of colored light has continued to this day.

One great benefit of colored light therapy is that, when used properly, it does not have any of the negative consequences and side effects that are often seen with conventional medical therapies, such as surgery and most medications.

The Research on Light Therapy

The history of light therapy is fascinating. Light therapy, particularly sunlight, has been in use since ancient times. In fact, in the early 1800's, physicians throughout the world believed that sunlight could cure a wide range of conditions, including inflammation, tuberculosis, and even paralysis. During this time, some studies even found that colored light produced dramatic effects on the brain and the nervous system. However, it wasn't until the 1870's that researchers began to look in earnest at the possible therapeutic benefits of colored light.

One of the pioneers in colored light therapy was General Augustus J. Pleasanton. In 1876, General Pleasanton reported that the use of blue light—from the sun or from an artificial source—was effective in stimulating the endocrine glands and nervous systems, both of which have significant effects on your mood, level of energy, and sleep patterns.

One year later, prominent physician Dr. Seth Pancoast filtered sunlight through panes of red or blue glass and found that this could either increase or decrease the activity of the nervous system, and that by these opposing colors, he could create emotional as well as physical balance in the body. More than a decade later, Dr. Niels Finsen took the treatment one step further and used red light to treat smallpox lesions.

Light Research in the Twentieth Century

All of these early pioneers paved the way for more intense research on colored light during the 20th century. In the early 1900's, Dr. Harry Spitler began researching this type of therapy to treat patients. By the 1920's, his research revealed that certain portions of the brain that directly control both the autonomic nervous system and the endocrine system are regulated, at least in part, by light.

He also discovered that light may play a very significant role in altering behavior and physiological function. In other words, simply altering the color of light entering the eyes could disturb or restore balance within the autonomic nervous system that regulates many physical functions including heart rate and muscle tension. In this way, light not only affects your emotional makeup and mood, but it can also have an impact on several physical functions, including energy and sleep.

This research focus progressed significantly in the 1950's, when Russian scientist, S.V. Krakov discovered that the color red stimulated the sympathetic portion of the autonomic nervous system, while the color blue stimulated the parasympathetic portion. In 1958, Dr. Robert Gerard confirmed this finding.

In Gerard's study, blue, red, and white lights of equal brightness were each projected separately for 10 minutes on a screen in front of 24 normal adult males. He found that red light stimulated the sympathetic nervous system, increasing the level of alertness, excitement, and tension in the subject, while the blue and white lights stimulated the parasympathetic nervous system and generated a sense of calm and relaxation.

Recent Research on Light Therapy

The effect of red light on greatly boosting energy was studied in more depth by the Russian biophysicist Tina Karu, Ph.D., of the Laser Technology Center in Moscow, She and her colleagues spent years studying these and other beneficial effects of red light therapy. She is one of the most renowned researchers on red light in the world, and I was thrilled to learn of her impressive and tremendously compelling body of research on red light.

Dr. Karu and other researchers made a landmark discovery in the way red light affects our bodies at the cellular level. Various wavelengths of red light easily penetrate the skin and stimulate energy production within the mitochondria, the energy-producing powerhouses of the cells. They enable the energy from food to be released and trapped as high-energy bonds called adenosine triphosphate (ATP). ATP is found in all of our cells and releases energy needed to fuel nearly all chemical reactions in our bodies. Thus, red light therapy helps your body create energy, vitality, and stamina, so every tissue and organ system can run more efficiently.

The Effect of Light Therapy on the Brain and Endocrine System

Colored light is absorbed into your body through your eyes or skin. When taken in through the eyes, colored light is converted into electrical impulses through the action of millions of cells that are sensitive to light and color. The electrical impulses move along the optical nerve to the hypothalamus gland in the brain, which regulates a variety of body functions including breathing, digestion, temperature, blood pressure, mood, and sexual function.

The stimulatory effect that light has on the hypothalamus then affects the hypothalamus's action on the pituitary gland. The pituitary controls the secretion of many hormones including those of your thyroid gland, the thymus gland that regulates immunity, your adrenal glands that support your energy and vitality as well as your ovaries that produce female reproductive hormones like estrogen and progesterone.

The pineal gland, located in the brain, also receives light waves through the eye, which are then transformed into nerve impulses capable of affecting hormones. This important gland regulates our sleep-wake patterns and, through the secretion of the brain hormone melatonin, promotes deep, peaceful restful sleep that is essential for energy and vitality. When taken in through the skin, colored light can penetrate up to one inch in the soft tissue. By traveling energetic pathways, light therapy has a therapeutic effect on the endocrine glands and other organ systems

One of the best-known and widely respected modern-day researchers of the effects of colored light on the brain and endocrine system is Dr. Norman Shealy, a neurosurgeon by training and a prominent practitioner of complementary medicine. He has taken the research on colored light therapy's effect on the brain one step further by actually incorporating light therapy into his practice, using flashing bright light and colored light to treat depression and pain. Dr. Shealy has found that stimulating colors like red and relaxing colors like blue and violet has an effect on many neurochemicals, neurotransmitters, and even hormones, including sex hormones.

The Healing Benefits of Red Light

In general, red light is profoundly anti-aging and promotes energy, strength, and vitality for virtually every organ in the body as well as relieving pain caused by many different types of conditions including fibromyalgia. It also reduces muddled thinking and poor mental acuity and increases mental clarity and sharpness in women with chronic fatigue. It has also been found to have a stimulatory effect on the pituitary and immune systems. We'll be looking at many of these benefits in this section!

Red Light and Chronic Fatigue and Tiredness

One of the most beneficial effects of red light is that it greatly boosts energy, strength and vitality. As I mentioned earlier in this book, Dr. Tina Karu and other researchers made a landmark discovery in the way red light affects our bodies at the cellular level.

Various wavelengths of red light easily penetrate the skin and stimulate energy production within the mitochondria, the energy-producing powerhouses of the cells. They enable the energy from food to be released and trapped as high-energy bonds called adenosine triphosphate (ATP). ATP is found in all of our cells and releases energy needed to fuel nearly all the chemical reactions in our bodies. Thus, red light therapy helps your body create energy, vitality, and stamina, so every tissue and organ system can run more efficiently.

Red light is tremendously beneficial for women suffering from chronic fatigue and tiredness because of its energizing effects.

Red Light and Hormone Health

Red light triggers sympathetic nervous system function, which increases your level of mental and physical energy, causes your heart and pulse rate to speed up and your body to get rid of excess fluids through increased urination. Plus, more calories are burned up and utilized for energy. It also has a stimulatory effect on brain and hormonal functions.

You may benefit from red light therapy if you are in menopause and suffer from lack of libido, energy, stamina, and poor mental acuity. Some postmenopausal women find that once their menstrual periods cease, their metabolism slows down and they gain weight more easily and become more sluggish in general. Red light therapy may help them to lose weight by speeding up their metabolism through the sympathetic nervous system. It has also been found to have a stimulatory effect on the pituitary and immune systems.

Red Light and Depression

Red light therapy has a stimulating and energizing effect on the brain and nervous system. It supports the production of brain chemicals that give us energy, vitality and zest for life including the excitatory neurotransmitters such as dopamine, epinephrine, and norepinephrine. For individuals whose brain chemistry and emotional patterns tends towards depression, feeling down or sad, using red light therapy can be helpful and uplifting. I have seen this beneficial effect of red light on mood in a number of women. The beneficial effects of red light trigger chemicals within the brain that also make us more positive, optimistic and more outwardly social.

A woman who is genuinely light deficient in the red light part of the electromagnetic spectrum may find that she needs to supplement with these light frequencies on an ongoing basis to feel her best and function well.

Red Light and Pain

Pain, discomfort and stiffness can occur due to disease, trauma, injury or overuse in various parts of the body. Chronic pain is very common and affects 47 percent of adults in the U.S. on an ongoing basis. Pain can be seen in people of all ages. I have had patients as young as the early and mid-twenties complain about chronic pain, often from sports injuries and illness, and patients in their eighties for whom pain was their main symptom of disease. Pain medication doesn't solve the problem and offers only symptom relief with, unfortunately, many unpleasant side effects ranging from gastrointestinal symptoms, addiction, and even kidney and liver failure with chronic overuse.

Happily, red light can be used alone or combined with infrared light therapy for the successful treatment of pain and can offer genuine relief for pain sufferers. While we cannot see infrared light the way we do colored visible light, we can feel its heating effects on the body. Infrared light penetrates deeply into the body, helping to improve circulation and increasing oxygenation, and immune enhancing blood cells to the area of injury. Like red light, it also stimulates the production of collagen.

When red light is used by itself or in combination with infrared, it has been found in research studies to provide relief of pain and discomfort in muscles, ligaments, tendons, burses, nerves, subcutaneous tissues, and even organs.

Red light therapy has been used to treat pain due to various causes for several decades with great results. These include fibromyalgia, migraine headaches, bursitis, carpel tunnel syndrome, osteoarthritis, muscle spasm and strains. Let's focus on the benefits of red light therapy for fibromyalgia.

Red Light Relieves Fibromyalgia

As discussed earlier in the book, if you suffer from fibromyalgia you are likely to have pain, chronic fatigue, sleep disturbances, muscle spasms, joint stiffness, difficulty concentrating, and mood symptoms such as depression or anxiety. Some patients even suffer from difficulty swallowing, irritable bowel and bladder, and numbness and tingling.

Unfortunately, it is a debilitating and difficult to treat condition. In addition, there is no definitive lab test to diagnose fibromyalgia and it is diagnosed by the process of elimination of other conditions.

Luckily, red light laser therapy offers significant benefits for the treatment and relief of fibromyalgia. In one study published in *Rheumatology International*, 75 fibromyalgia patients were divided into three groups that were treated daily for eight weeks with either cold red light laser, "fake" laser (the control), or the commonly prescribed fibromyalgia medication amitriptyline.

During the study, these patients were being monitored for changes in pain, number of tender points, fatigue, tenderness of skin folds, muscle spasms, sleep, morning stiffness, depression, and quality-of-life scores from a standardized fibromyalgia test. Results of this study showed that the cold red light laser group had significant improvement across the board and experienced excellent relief from pain, fatigue, and morning stiffness.

In another study published in *Lasers in Medical Science*, women with fibromyalgia were divided into two groups and treated daily for two weeks with either a cold red light laser or a "fake" laser. The cold red light laser group had superior improvement in pain, muscle spasm, morning stiffness, and a number of tender points.

Red light therapy also provides tremendous relief from the pain and stiffness associated with fibromyalgia. Colored light from red light LEDs (light-emitting diodes) and near infrared (NIR) penetrates as deep as an inch through the skin and into soft tissue, and it is well documented to accelerate healing, increase cellular metabolism and energy production, and relieve pain and stiffness as reported in *Photomedicine and Laser Surgery*.

Finally, in a randomized, controlled study published in *Lasers in Medical Science* that followed 64 volunteers, researchers found that red light LED's and infrared therapy used in combination relieved pain by normalizing activated nerve fibers. This is particularly relevant for the hypersensitive nerve reactions so commonly found in patients with fibromyalgia.

To treat fibromyalgia, I recommend that you apply red light LED's directly over each painful area for one to 15 minutes. Cold laser red light therapy can be also used to treat your tender points.

Applying Colored Light to the Body

In addition to regular exposure to natural sunlight, you can use colored light in three different ways: lasers (which are mainly used for red light therapy), light-emitting diodes (LEDs), or a colored glass or gel filter. Unlike the light bulbs we use in our homes and offices that radiate light throughout the room and are made of many colors, lasers travel as a single beam in one direction and are made up of a single color. Traditionally, there have been red light lasers, though new lasers are now becoming available that utilize other parts of the color spectrum. For example, blue lasers are effective for mood and brain function, while violet is great for treating infection, including dental-related infectious issues such as gum infections, cavities, and root canal infections, as well as infectious diseases in general.

Lasers comprise one of the fastest growing areas of energy medicine. They offer amazing versatility, and can be extremely beneficial for a wide range of conditions, including menstrual and hormonal issues, cancer, soft tissue injury, brain and neurological diseases, emotional imbalances, and macular degeneration.

Don't confuse these types of lasers with the "hot" lasers used by surgeons to cut, cauterize, and destroy tissue. Light-therapy lasers have a powerful regenerative and healing effect upon many different types of sick or injured tissues. They use coherent energy, which is the same energy used by the cells in your body to communicate to one another. This is one of the reasons lasers are the most efficient energy your body can use to regenerate tissue and increase blood flow.

Plus, research is showing that the coherent energy of lasers helps to stimulate the nervous system. This is an exciting area that we are learning more and more about every day. While these types of lasers are generally safe, they have traditionally been used by health care professionals (although wonderful red lasers have now become available for self-care use at home and are tremendously helpful).

Specific wavelengths of light can also be transmitted through LEDs, which is an excellent method for women who want to use colored light therapy on a self-care basis. Each diode is very small; in fact, the red LEDs that have been used by NASA to promote wound healing of astronauts are no larger than a pinhead. But when linked together, these diodes form a flat panel of colored light that produces a beam that is broader than that of a laser.

Unlike a laser, specific wavelengths of LEDs can be used simultaneously with other colored light bands to expand their therapeutic benefits. The great thing about LEDs is that the light they emit is completely safe and can be used on such sensitive areas as the eyes. Plus, they are much safer to use than lasers, can be bought by anyone, and are readily available for purchase.

The third way colored light is transmitted is through a simple, filtered light. This form of light therapy was practiced in ancient times, and today involves placing a red glass or theatrical gel filter over a common light bulb or a full-spectrum fluorescent bulb, or even in glasses or a contact lens!

Self-Treating With Colored Light

Colored light can be placed on many different parts of your body. I prefer the area three finger-widths below the navel. You can also use your "third eye" — the point directly between your eyebrows, where the bridge of your nose meets your eyebrows — or the area in the center of your breastbone, at the level of your heart. However, you should avoid this area if you have a pacemaker or known heart disease.

Treatment sessions can last anywhere from just a few minutes to as long as 15 minutes (or even longer if appropriate), depending on what feels most comfortable to you. Not all women need or should use prolonged light therapy. Start out by using any light therapy device for shorter amounts of time (just a minute or two) in the beginning until you know how your body will respond.

If you find that you enjoy colored light therapy and want to use it as part of your regular health program, it is important to be aware that your emotions and level of energy will likely change as you move through different life stages. As this occurs, you may find that you need to modify your colored light program.

Red light devices including red light LEDs, red light lasers and even colored glasses with red lenses are readily available for purchase through the Internet. Even Amazon.com markets a wide variety of red light LED devices, including light devices for the relief of pain!

Colored light therapy is extremely safe; however, I suggest that you consult the manufacturer of the light unit you purchase to see if there are any contra-indications between your condition and their particular product.

Bright Light Therapy for Fatigue and Depression

Many women with chronic fatigue feel worse during the winter months. Along with fatigue, they often notice a deepening depression, weight gain, lowered body temperature, difficulty awakening in the morning, daytime drowsiness, and an increased craving for sweets. People affected with these symptoms tend to withdraw socially and experience a drop in their work performance.

Researchers who have studied this problem over the past few decades call it Seasonal Affective Disorder (or by its acronym, SAD); they have found that it is triggered by the decreased hours of daylight in winter. Interestingly, they also learned that the problem is worse in northern latitudes, where the level of light decreases even more in winter. The prevalence of SAD symptoms, not surprisingly, ranges from 1 to 2 percent in Florida to 10 percent in Alaska.

Scientists believe that a deficiency of daylight causes depression by altering the rhythms of our daily biological processes, called circadian rhythms, and by delaying nightly secretions of melatonin, a hormone involved in the regulation of sleep. Those who suffer from SAD may also have disturbances in production of other chemicals that carry messages from one brain cell to another, such as dopamine and serotonin. Research studies suggest that vision also plays a role in causing SAD. Some women's eyes are less light sensitive and therefore less capable of taking in light efficiently during short winter days.

Women with SAD often spend more time indoors in winter, living and working under dim incandescent light or fluorescent lights, which lack the full range of outdoor sunlight. These women may greatly benefit from a daily one-hour walk in normal winter sunlight, since they will receive the aerobic benefits as well as the additional light exposure. Moreover, daily exposure to artificial bright light that simulates daylight for a week or two in the winter appears to be a powerful treatment for chronic fatigue and depression. Many people treated with this technique have had dramatic relief of their symptoms.

The best units provide 10,000 lux of bright indoor lighting. (In contrast, sunshine produces 100,000 lux.) The light spectrum used in this product provides minimal exposure to the more harmful ultraviolet and blue rays and tends to emphasize the red rays, which have a mood-elevating effect. The box is positioned one to three feet away from the user, who is free to exercise, read, or work. People using these units generally find that 30 minutes of exposure each day, preferably in the morning, is all that's needed to improve mood and reduce SAD symptoms. Certain individuals require longer exposure, up to two hours. These light units are readily available through the Internet.

Chloe's Story

By the time Chloe came to me for help, she was 49 years old and had spent two perfectly miserable winters suffering from SAD. During her initial consultation, she told me that she had always had a tendency towards feeling mildly depressed, particularly during the week or so before her menstrual periods (when she suffered from PMS). She reported that when she entered menopause at age 47, she began to notice a worsening fatigue during the winter months.

As the days grew shorter, she had trouble just getting out of bed. She felt exhausted, "blue" and less sociable. She didn't feel "up" for anything, including her normal exercise routine. Come spring, she observed, the symptoms reversed, only to have the cycle repeat the next winter.

Chloe had read about the connection between light deprivation and mood before coming to see me. She wondered if she might be suffering from SAD — and was determined not to spend another winter feeling blue.

I suggested that she buy a light unit designed to treat SAD. The results exceeded Chloe's expectations. The way she described it, the light treatments were like a "cushion" that prevented her from sinking into depression.

That first winter with the light unit was the best Chloe had experienced in years. Using the light unit didn't just relieve her symptoms; it put her back in control of her life.

13

Physical Exercise for Relief of Chronic Fatigue

Many women with chronic fatigue simply stop exercising entirely because they lack the stamina and endurance to continue their habitual routines. I have seen in my practice many fit patients who were once regular joggers, bicyclists, or tennis players, but who stopped their activities altogether with the onset of chronic fatigue. Often these women became totally sedentary because their regular physical activities seemed to deplete their energy reserve.

This change from an active, athletic lifestyle to virtual inactivity is actually unhealthy. Movement is the wellspring of life. Without the pulsation of the cells, the beating of the heart, and the contraction of the muscles, life ceases. Lack of exercise reduces circulation and oxygenation to vital organs, such as the brain and heart, and reduces the metabolism of all the cells of the body that are needed for energy.

On the other hand, women with chronic fatigue shouldn't be doing a prolonged, strenuous workout, since this will deplete the available oxygen and fuel supply of their muscles, making them feel more tired than ever. Thus, jogging, fast dancing, vigorous bodybuilding, and a hard game of tennis are not desirable activities for women with chronic fatigue.

An optimal exercise program for chronic fatigue includes slower, gentler activities that promote muscle and joint flexibility, reduce stiffness and muscle tension, and help increase good blood circulation and oxygenation to the entire body. The possibilities include walking, stretching, deep breathing exercises, range of motion and flexibility exercises, and gentle swimming to help keep a woman fit without stressing the body to the point of exhaustion.

It is important to monitor your tolerance for exercise and increase the amount of exercise that you do to your fitness level. Women in the healing phase of chronic fatigue should never overdo any physical activity. Exercise should make you feel better, more energized, not more tired. Even if you need to start with just walking a small distance like a block or less, it is important to continue doing this on a regular basis, at least every other day or every day for even a few minutes to start. Over time, you will build up your exercise tolerance and your level of stamina and energy will begin to improve.

For example, if you find that walking a mile makes you too tired, try walking half that distance. If your fatigue is really severe and you are housebound for a period of time, then just doing deep breathing and flexibility exercises and even walking around the rooms of your house or your yard will be helpful. It is important to just keep moving to assist in your recovery.

If your pain is too great because of a condition like fibromyalgia, consider doing gentle range of motion exercises such as tilting your head from side to side and or rocking your hips from side to side. These exercises will help to loosen up your muscles.

Exercise of any type, especially moderate aerobic exercise like walking, will help to keep you from feeling too depressed and blue. Many of my chronic fatigue patients have complained of really low moods that hampered their quality of life and their effectiveness in solving the underlying health problems.

Unfortunately, inactivity has a depressant effect on mood. When my patients started to exercise regularly, their energy and mood picked up. In fact, many of them have found so much benefit in physical exercise as a way to reduce chronic fatigue and depression that it often has become their most effective form of stress management. They found that exercise produced a sense of peace and well-being unmatched by almost anything else that they did.

With regular aerobic exercise, you greatly improve blood flow and oxygenation to the brain, which in turn increases the production of beta-endorphins, the body's natural painkillers that give you a sense of euphoria and well-being and also reduces pain. It also helps promote other components of healthy brain chemistry, including the production of female hormones. By improving circulation, exercise facilitates proper nutrient flow and waste product removal.

The research on the benefits of exercise for energy and mood is very strong. While you may be familiar with this concept of exercise alleviating depression, you may not know that research has shown that it's as effective as commonly prescribed antidepressants.

According to a study from the *Archives of Medicine*, exercise was found to be as effective as medication in reducing depression among patients with major depression. Researchers randomly separated more than 150 men and women over the age of 50 with major depressive disorder into three groups. One group was given the antidepressant Zoloft (sertraline), the second group either rode a stationary bicycle, walked, or jogged for 30 minutes three times a week, and the third group received the antidepressant as well as the exercise regimen. All subjects underwent extensive evaluations for depression. After 16 weeks, researchers found that there was equal improvement in depressive levels between the groups.

A study from the *American Journal of Epidemiology* took these findings one-step further and set out to determine if exercise could actually prevent depression. Researchers studied nearly 2,000 adults aged 50 to 94 for more than 5 years, and rated their physical activity on an eight-point scale; with eight indicating the highest level of physical activity (activities included walking and swimming). They found that every one-point increase in activity lowered a person's risk of being depressed by 10 percent, and cut their risk of becoming depressed by 17 percent. Researchers concluded that physical activity did indeed have a protective effect on depression for older adults.

Exercise is also extremely useful in relieving the symptoms of fibromyalgia. In fact, a study published in the *Journal Arthritis and Rheumatism* found that women with fibromyalgia who participated in a strength training and walking program for 20 weeks improved their muscle strength, endurance, and overall ability to function without aggravating their symptoms.

In a review of 16 trials involving 724 fibromyalgia patients (Cochrane Database of Systematic Reviews); supervised aerobic exercise significantly improved aerobic performance, generalized pain, and tender point pain. Good types of exercise included swimming, water aerobics, biking as well as walking.

I want to share with you a few tips to make your walking program more enjoyable and beneficial:

Invest in a good pair of comfortable shoes. I recently discovered a wonderful brand of shoes made just for women - Rykä. Their shoes take into account women's narrower heels and wider forefoot, and offer lots of cushioning and support. Rykä can be found in most Lady Foot Lockers or ordered online at www.ryka.com.

Stretch before and after each walk. Take a few minutes to loosen up your legs, arms, back, and shoulders before and after each walking session. This is very important if you have a condition like fibromyalgia in which stiffness and muscle tightness are so prevalent.

Exercise outside as much as the weather allows. Take time to rejoice in nature and the change of the seasons. Note the way the grass smells after your neighbors have cut their lawn. Take in the red and orange foliage of autumn. Listen for the crunch of snow underfoot and the crispness of the winter air. Finally, inhale the aroma of new spring flowers. This will help to stimulate your brain in a beneficial way for restoring your level of energy. If the weather doesn't allow for outside activity, move your routine to a nearby mall or gently and slowly try the treadmill at a nearby gym.

As I previously mentioned, never rest on your laurels when doing an exercise program to restore you energy. In order to avoid plateauing, be sure to slowly build upon each success according to your tolerance level. If you start off walking for 10 to 15 minutes a day three days a week, try gradually building to 20 to 30 minutes a day 4 or 5 days a week; work towards a goal of eventually walking for one hour a day, 5 to 7 days a week.

In this chapter, I also share with you a sequence of easy to follow exercises that you can use in your self-care program to improve your vitality, flexibility and promote a sense of emotional well-being. You may want to combine them with moderate, aerobic exercises such as walking. You can also combine them with the stretches and acupressure massage points that I have also included further on in this book.

Guidelines for Physical Exercise

An exercise program for women with chronic fatigue, of necessity, must be gentle and not make too many demands on the body. Too strenuous an exercise program can leave a woman feeling more exhausted than ever. Therefore, I have included in this program only routines that promote blood flow and oxygenation to the vital organs as well as the muscles, decrease muscle stiffness and tension, and help loosen the joints. Since depression and chronic fatigue frequently co-exist, I have included mood-elevating exercises that can help you regain the zest for life that so many women with chronic fatigue feel is missing. You may also find these exercises helpful during times of increased emotional stress and tension.

Before you begin the exercise program for chronic fatigue; read through the following guidelines. These will allow you to perform the exercises in an optimal manner and without creating undue stress.

- Do all of these exercises during the first week or two of your program. Try the exercises that most appeal to you, then put together your own routine. You may find that you want to use all of them on a regular basis, or perhaps only a few. You can use any of these as warm-ups before participating in sports or athletic events.

- Perform the exercises in a relaxed and unhurried manner. Be sure to set aside adequate time—15 to 30 minutes—so that you don't feel rushed. Your exercise area should be quiet, peaceful, and uncluttered.

- Choose a flat area and work on a mat or a blanket. This will make you more comfortable while you do the exercises.

- Wear loose, comfortable clothing. It is better to exercise without socks to give your feet complete freedom of movement and to prevent slipping.

- Wait at last two hours after eating to exercise. Evacuate your bowels or bladder before you begin the exercises.

- Pay close attention to the initial instructions when beginning an exercise. Look at the placement of the body as shown in the photographs. This is very important, for you are much more likely to get relief from your symptoms if you practice the exercise properly.

- Try to visualize the exercise in your mind, then follow with proper placement of the body.

- Move slowly through the exercise. This will help promote flexibility of the muscles and prevent injury.

- Always rest for a few minutes after doing the exercises.

- Try to practice these movements on a regular basis. A short session every day is best. If that is not possible, then try to practice them every other day.

Exercise 1: Deep Breathing

Deep, slow abdominal breathing is essential for women with chronic fatigue. It expands your lungs and allows you to bring adequate oxygen, the fuel for metabolic activity, to all the tissues of your body. Rapid, shallow breathing decreases your oxygen supply and keeps you tired and devitalized. Deep breathing helps to relax the entire body and strengthens the muscles in the chest and abdomen. It helps to stabilize mood and reduce both depression and anxiety, so it is very important for emotional well-being.

Lie flat on your back with your knees pulled up. Keep your feet slightly apart. Try to breathe in and out through your nose.

Inhale deeply. As you breathe in, allow your stomach to relax so that the air flows into your abdomen. Your stomach should balloon out as you breathe in. Visualize your lungs filling up with air so that your chest swells out.

Imagine that the air you breathe is filling your body with energy.

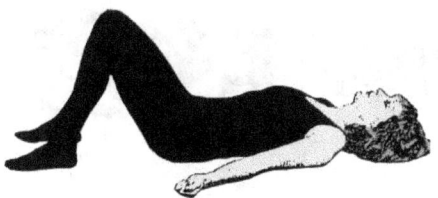

Exhale deeply. As you breathe out, let your stomach and chest collapse. Imagine the air being pushed out, first from your abdomen and then from your lungs.

Exercise 2: Total Body Muscle Relaxation

Women with chronic fatigue tend to have poor muscle tone. They frequently have muscle groups that are tense and tight because of inadequate oxygenation and blood flow. Lactic acid tends to accumulate in these muscles, and muscle tension can become a chronic problem. Regular physical activity effectively breaks up this pattern of chronically tight muscles. Unfortunately, women with chronic fatigue tend to become less active as their tiredness worsens. Although strenuous exercise is often too difficult for a woman with chronic fatigue, it is still very important to keep the muscles loose and flexible. Supple muscles have a beneficial effect on mood and induce a sense of peace and calm. The following exercise helps you to get in touch with the parts of your body that feel tense and contracted. It will also aid in releasing muscle tension.

Lie in a comfortable position. Allow your arms to rest limply, palms down, on the surface next to you. Breathe slowly and deeply as you do this exercise.

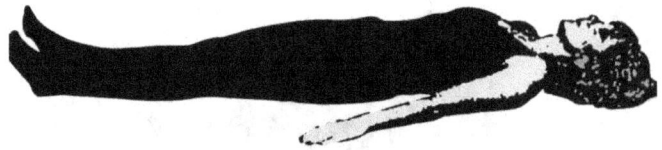

Raise your right hand off the floor and hold it there for 15 seconds. Notice any tension in your forearm or upper arm. Let your hand slowly relax and rest on the floor. The hand and arm muscles should relax. As you lie there, notice any other parts of your body where you are carrying tension.

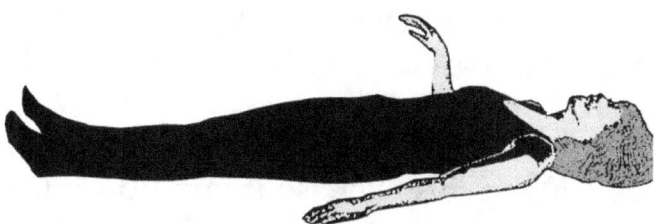

Clench your hands into fists and hold them closed for 15 seconds, then let your hands relax.

Now, tense and relax the following parts of your body in this order: face, shoulders, back, stomach, pelvis, legs, feet, and toes. Hold each part tensed for 15 seconds and then relax your body for 30 seconds before going on to the next part.

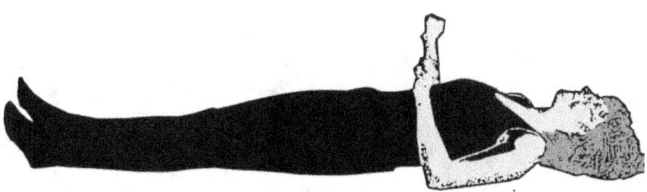

Visualize the tense part contracting and becoming tighter. On relaxing, see the energy flowing into the entire body like a gentle wave, making all the muscles soft and pliable.

Finish the exercise by shaking your hands. Imagine the remaining tension flowing out of your fingertips.

Exercise 3: Energizing Sequence

This exercise sequence is excellent for increasing your energy, releasing muscle tension, and improving circulation. Many women feel increased vitality and vigor upon completing this set. The exercise stimulates movement and energy flow through all muscles of the body, starting from the legs and moving up to the top of the head. These exercises are based on traditional energy healing models in which these exercises are thought to stimulate the major chakras or vital energy centers of the body.

Do the steps in this sequence slowly, to avoid stressing the body. You will better feel the benefits of this exercise if you don't rush through the steps or do them too hard. As your strength and flexibility improve, you may want to do the steps a little more vigorously.

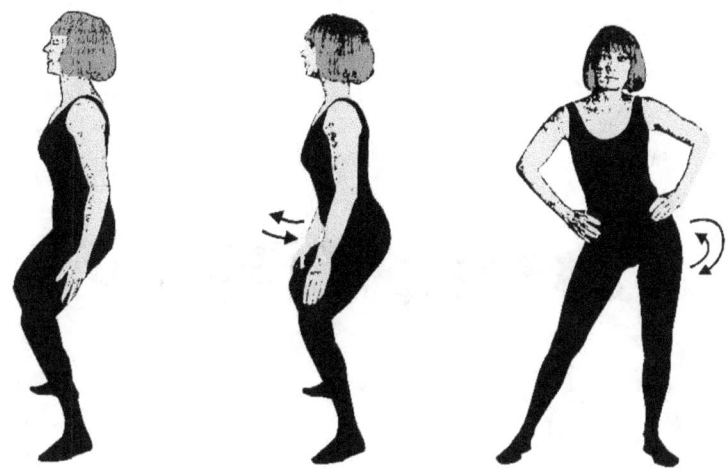

Stand with your legs spread apart about 2 feet. Point your feet out at a comfortable angle.

Rock your pelvis back and forth

Repeat 10 times. Then rotate your hips in a circular fashion, first moving clockwise and then counterclockwise.

Pelvis and Lower Abdomen

Lie on your stomach, placing your fists under your hips. Rest your forehead on the floor.

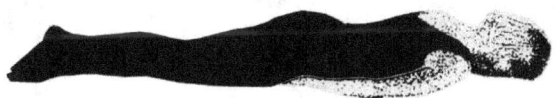

As you inhale, raise your right leg with an upward thrust, keeping your hips on your fists. Hold for 5 to 20 seconds if possible.

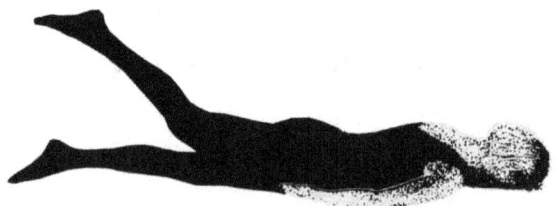

Lower the leg and slowly bring it back to the original position.

Repeat several times. Then do the exercise on the left side.

Abdomen and Chest

Sit on your heels with your hands placed on your knees. As you inhale, arch your back and stretch to expand your chest up and out.

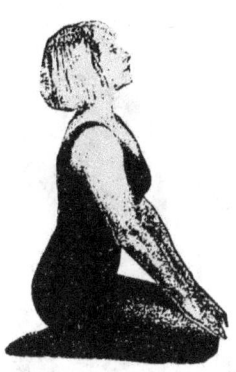

As you exhale, slump down to curve you back

Repeat several times.

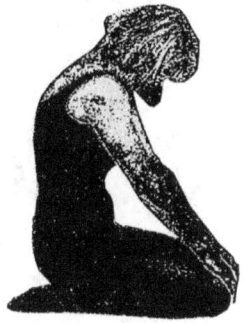

Abdomen and Shoulders

Sit on the floor with your legs out in front. Raise your arms to shoulder level, bending them at the elbow.

Place your hands on your shoulders with your fingers in front and thumbs in back.

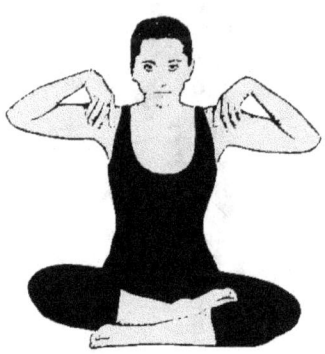

Turn your elbows, head, and neck to the left and then to the right.

Repeat 10 times. Be sure to let your entire torso move with your shoulders and arms.

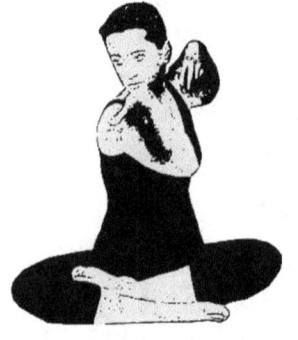 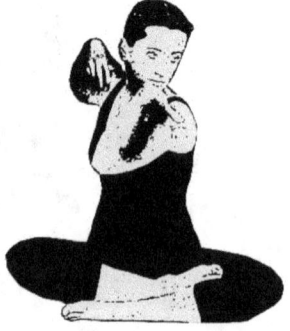

Lean backward over a hassock or a big soft pillow, so that your chest opens and expands as your shoulders go backward.

Let the muscles of your chest relax.

Keep your feet firmly on the floor.

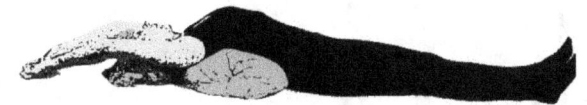

Neck

Sit on your knees with your hands on your thighs. Take a deep breath and stretch your body upward.

As you exhale, widen your eyes, stick out your tongue and push your body forward. Hold this position to the count of 10.

Repeat this exercise 5 times.

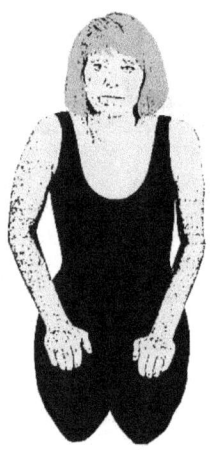
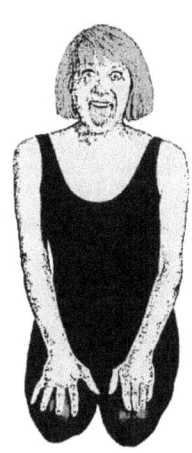

Then lie flat on your back on the floor in a relaxed manner.

As you inhale, slowly turn your head to the left. Then, exhale as you return your head to the center position.

As you inhale again, turn your head to the right. Continue this exercise for 1 minute.

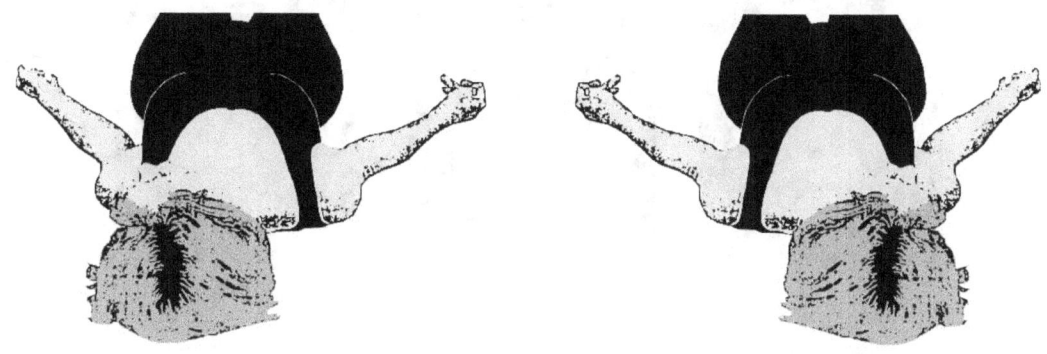

Eyes

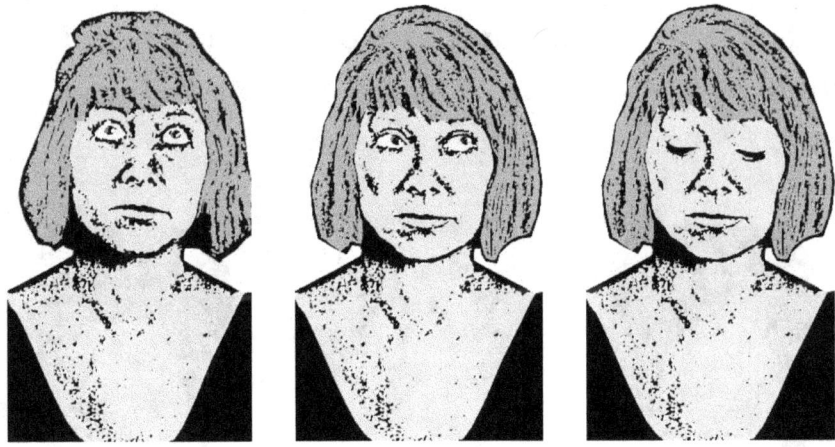

With your head facing straight and your facial muscles relaxed, roll your eye muscles in the following directions: up and down, and side to side.

Move your eye muscles up to the left and down to the right.

Reverse, moving your eyes up to the right and down to the left.

Head

Lie on your back. Your arms should be at your sides, palms up.

Close your eyes and relax your whole body.

Inhale and exhale slowly, breathing from the diaphragm.

Rub the crown of your head in a clockwise motion with your right hand for 30 seconds.

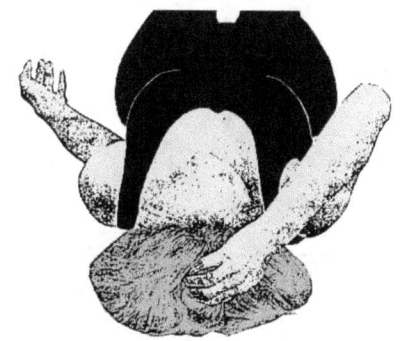

Activity Chart for Chronic Fatigue

Lower body exercise:	Walking
Upper body exercise:	Weight lifting (low impact)
Whole body exercise:	Swimming Ballroom dancing Golf
Flexibility exercise:	Stretches T'ai chi

Benefits of Exercise

- Improves oxygenation and blood circulation to the entire body.

- Improves functions of vital organs, including nervous system and digestive tract.

- Improves flexibility and decreases joint and muscle stiffness.

- Relieves depression, insomnia, anxiety, and irritability.

- Improves physical stamina and endurance.

- Increases your vigor and energy.

14

Stretches for Relief of Chronic Fatigue

Many different stretches can improve your level of energy and vitality while you're healing from chronic fatigue. Practiced slowly and gently, these exercises can provide many physiological and emotional benefits for your body. A good stretching routine stretches every muscle in the body, promoting limberness and flexibility in the muscles and joints. At the same time, better circulation and oxygenation to the whole body stimulates metabolism and improves cell function.

Improving circulation and nutrient flow to the brain and nervous system promotes healthy brain chemistry. This helps improve your mood, relieve depression, and reduce fatigue. Best of all, stretching is such an easy and gentle form of exercise that it can be practiced by most people, even women with severe chronic fatigue. Stretching is one of the few forms of physical activity that will not tire out a woman who has low physical reserve and stamina. When practiced on a regular basis, a good stretching routine can be an important part of your self-help program to regain your vigor and vitality.

When doing the exercises, it is important that you focus and concentrate on the positions. First your mind visualizes how the exercise is to look, and then your body follows with the correct placement of the pose. The exercises are done through slow, controlled stretching movements. This slowness enables you to have greater control over your body movements. You minimize the possibility of injury and maximize the benefit to the particular part of the body you are stretching. Follow the breathing instructions provided in the exercise. Most important, do not hold your breath. Allow your breath to flow in and out easily and effortlessly.

When beginning an exercise, pay close attention to the initial instructions. Look at the placement of the body as shown in the photographs. This is very important, because if you practice the pose properly, you are much more likely to get relief from your symptoms.

If you practice these stretches regularly in a slow, unhurried fashion, you will gradually loosen your muscles, ligaments, and joints. You may be surprised at how supple you can become over time. If you experience any discomfort, you have probably overreached your current ability and should immediately reduce the amount of the stretching until you can proceed without discomfort.

If you have any limitation or injury in any part of your body that would make it difficult to do a particular stretch (or set of stretches), they should be avoided. Only do those stretches that look comfortable to you to do and that you enjoy doing.

Stretch 1

This exercise helps relieve fatigue by releasing tension in the shoulder blades. Tension in the shoulders blocks blood flow and oxygenation to the head and neck area, making you feel mentally tired and sluggish.

Stand easily with your legs apart. As you exhale, drop your head and body slowly forward.

Let your fingers hang down as close to the ground as possible. Deep breathe in this position for 30 seconds.

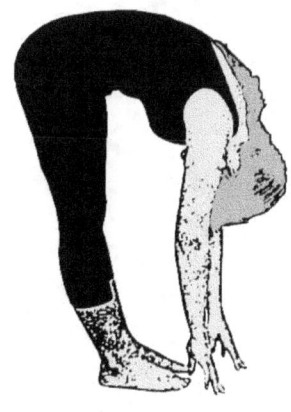

Slowly come up to the standing position.

Repeat 3 times.

Stretch 2

This exercise increases circulation to the upper half of the body, energizing and stimulating the body. It also loosens and stretches tense muscles in the upper body, especially the shoulders and back, and expands the lungs.

Stand easily. Arms should be at your sides; feet are hip distance apart.

Extend your arms forward until your palms touch.

Bring your arms back slowly and gracefully until you can clasp them behind your back.

Exhale, then straighten your clasped hands and arms as far as you can without discomfort. Remember to stand upright; body should not bend forward. Breathe deeply into chest.

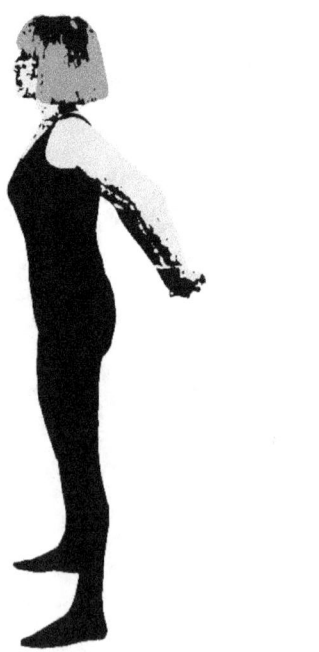 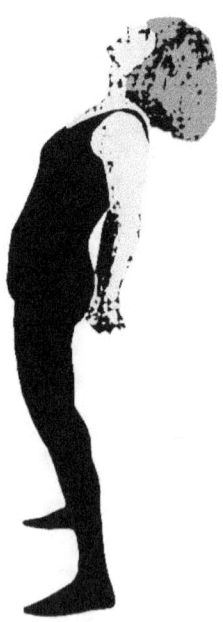

As you hold your breath, bend forward at the waist, bringing your clasped hands and arms up over your back.

Relax your neck muscles and keep your knees straight. Hold for a few seconds.

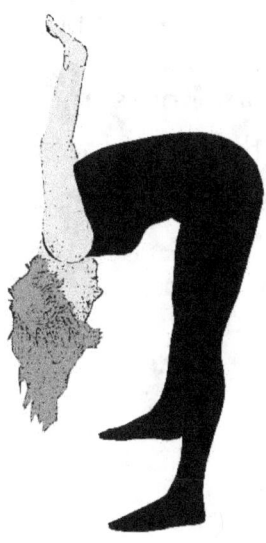

Exhale as you return to the upright position. Unclasp your hands and allow your arms to rest easily at your sides.

Repeat entire sequence 3 times.

Stretch 3

This exercise massages the entire neck, spine, and back muscles, as well as all the acupressure points along the spine. It will help to stimulate a sluggish thyroid by stretching and massaging the neck. This exercise will invigorate and energize you, reducing fatigue.

Lie on your back. Bend and raise your knees to your chest, clasping them with your hands. Hands should be interlocked above knees.

Raise your head toward your knees and gently rock back and forth on your curved spine. Note the roundness of your back and shoulders. Keep the chin tucked in as you roll back. Avoid rolling back too far on your neck.

Rock back and forth 5 to 10 times.

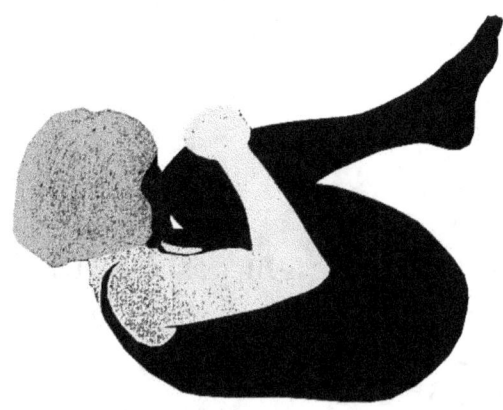

Stretch 4

This exercise helps to release overall body tension. It improves circulation and concentration. It helps to strengthen the lower back and abdominal area.

Lie on your stomach with your feet together and your arms lying flat at your sides.

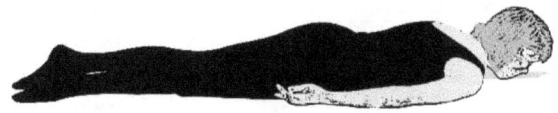

Stretch your arms out straight in front of you on the floor.

As you inhale, arch your back and lift your arms, head, chest, and legs off the floor. Hold the pose as long as you can, up to 30 seconds, breathing deeply and slowly.

Return to the original resting position with your head turned to the side, and completely relax for 1 to 3 minutes.

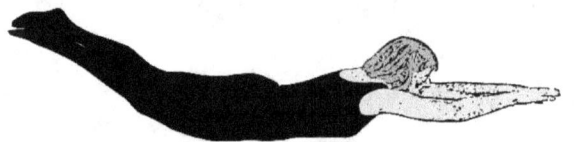

Stretch 5

This exercise helps relieve PMS fatigue and other premenstrual and menopausal symptoms by energizing the female reproductive tract. It also energizes the liver, intestines, and kidneys. It strengthens the lower back, abdomen, buttocks, and legs.

Lie face down on the floor. Make fists with both your hands and place them under your hips. This prevents compression of the lumbar spine while doing the exercise.

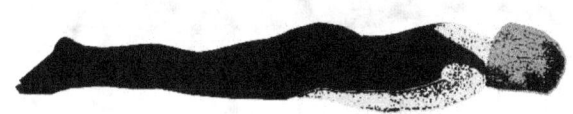

Straighten your body and raise your right leg with an upward thrust as high as you can, keeping your hips on your fists. Hold for 5 to 20 seconds if possible.

Lower the leg and slowly return to your original position. Repeat with the left leg, then with both legs together. Remember to keep your hips resting on your fists.

Repeat 10 times.

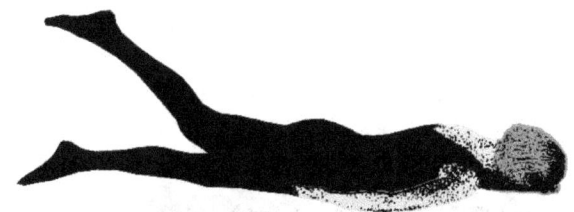

Stretch 6

This exercise is one of the most powerful stretches for increasing total body energy and vitality and releasing muscle tension. It strengthens the nervous system, improves concentration and mental clarity, and relieves depression. It also stimulates the thyroid, thymus, liver, kidney, and female reproductive tract. It helps to improve digestive function and may reduce sugar craving.

Lie face down on the floor, arms at your sides.

Slowly bend your legs at the knees and bring your feet up toward your buttocks.

Reach back with your arms and carefully take hold of first one foot and then the other. Flex your feet to make grasping them easier.

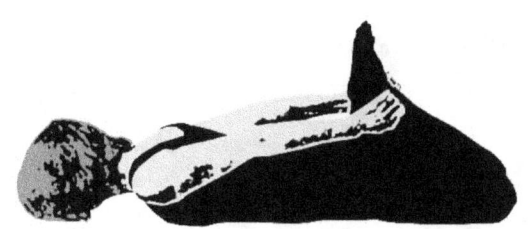

As you inhale, lift your head and raise your trunk from the floor as far as possible. Bring your knees together and lift your legs off the floor as far as possible, too. Imagine your body looking like a gently curved bow. Hold for 10 to 15 seconds.

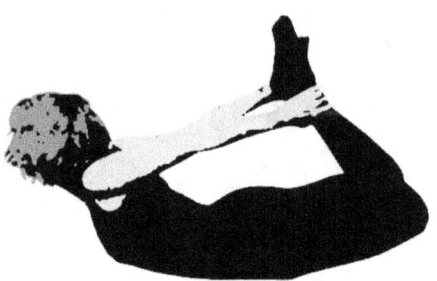

Slowly release the posture. Allow your chin to touch the floor and finally release your feet and return them slowly to the floor. Return to your original position.

Repeat 5 times.

Stretch 7

This exercise is used in the practice of yoga to improve your resistance to infections. It is thought to help prevent colds and respiratory infections, to reduce the duration of a cold, or to relieve allergic and respiratory symptoms.

Lie on your back with your knees bent and the bottoms of your feet flat on the floor.

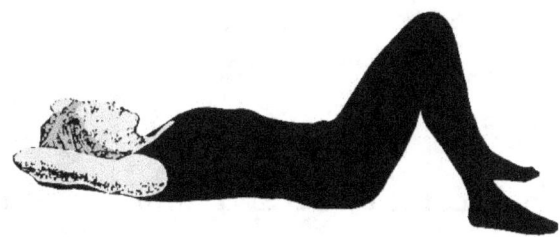

Bring your hands under your neck with the backs of your hands pressing against each other and the knuckles of your smallest fingers pressing into the base of your skull. Spread your index finger and thumb apart on each hand.

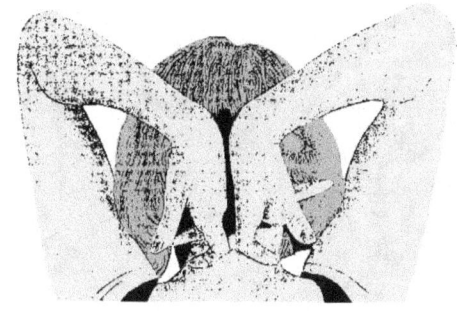

Inhale deeply and arch your hips up. Breathe deeply in this position for up to 1 minute.

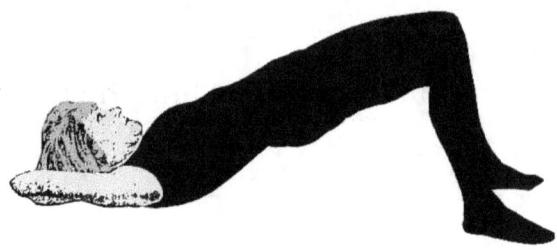

As you exhale, slowly come down and return to your original position.

Relax in this position for 1 to 3 minutes.

Stretch 8

This exercise is also thought to help increase resistance to infections, particularly colds and flu, as well as decrease fatigue. It also helps clear tension around the shoulder blades.

Sit on your heels, placing the instep of one foot into the arch of the other.

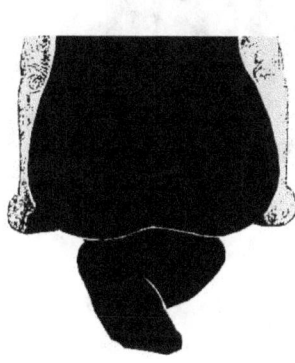

Lower your head slowly forward to the ground, bringing your arms behind your back and interlocking your fingers. Be sure to have your palms facing each other.

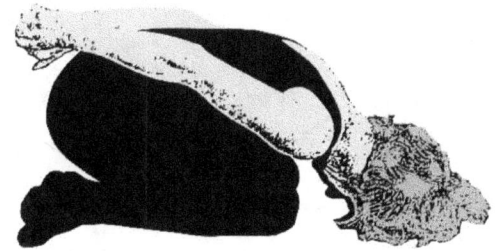

As you inhale, raise your arms straight up, keeping your hands clasped together.

Hold this position for up to 1 minute, breathing deeply.

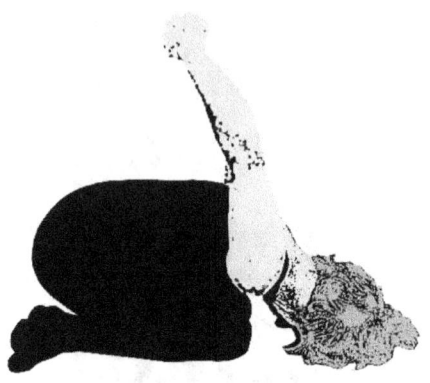

As you exhale, slowly unclasp your hands and let your arms relax on the floor, palms up.

Relax in this position for 1 to 3 minutes.

Stretch 9

This exercise helps relieve emotional tension and frustration. By helping release emotional upset locked in the muscles, side rolls promote a sense of mental balance and improved energy and vitality.

Lie on your back with your hands interlaced under your neck. As you inhale, bend and lift your right leg.

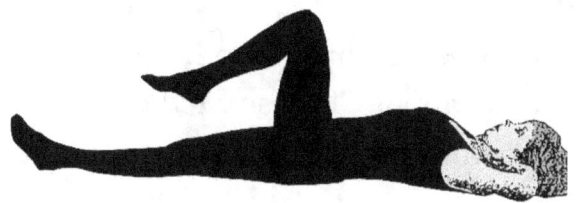

Then exhale and roll on your left side, with your knee touching the ground. As you do this, release a sigh.

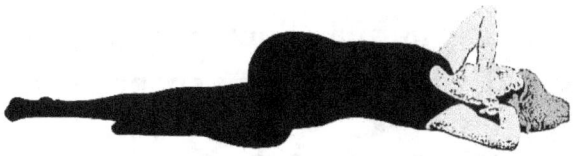

As you inhale, return to your original position. Repeat this 10 times, alternating sides. Then relax on your back for 1 minute.

15

Acupressure for Relief of Chronic Fatigue

Acupressure is an effective technique of Chinese massage that has traditionally been used to relieve chronic fatigue and improve energy, stamina, and endurance. Specific points on the skin are stimulated through gentle finger pressure that benefits energy levels. On the physical level, acupressure massage improves blood circulation, muscle tension, and other physiological functions. On a more subtle level, acupressure is believed to release the body's supply of life energy to fight disease and promote healing. In Traditional Chinese Medicine, this life energy is called chi; it is in some ways similar to electromagnetic energy.

The chi is thought to run through the body in channels called meridians. When flowing freely, the chi moves through the meridians throughout the whole body, sometimes on the surface of the skin and sometimes deep inside the body, in the organs. Health occurs only when the chi is present in sufficient amounts and is equally distributed throughout the body, energizing all organ systems. When the energy flow in a meridian is stopped or blocked, disease occurs. Thus, acupressure massage is based on the belief that effective therapy restores and balances the body's energy. Stimulating the acupressure points on the skin surface corrects the meridian flow. When the normal flow of energy through the body is restored, the body is believed to heal itself spontaneously.

You can perform acupressure massage on yourself, or a friend can do it. Unlike acupuncture, acupressure does not require the use of needles, so it is safe, painless, and doesn't require years of specialized training. For years, my patients have been very pleased with the results of using acupressure on specific points. Try the points mentioned in this chapter for relief of chronic fatigue and tiredness. You may find that acupressure massage is an important part of your personal self-help program.

Guidelines for Acupressure

Before you begin the acupressure exercises, read through the following guidelines. These guidelines will help you do the exercises correctly and make sure you receive the maximum benefit from them. I recommend that you try all the acupressure exercises during your first few treatment sessions. Then choose those that seem to benefit you the most and practice them on a regular basis.

- Try acupressure when you are relaxed. Make the room warm and quiet. Wash your hands and trim your nails to avoid bruising yourself. If your hands are cold, warm them in water.

- Work on the side of the body that has the most discomfort. If both sides are equally uncomfortable, choose whichever side you want. Working on one side seems to relieve the symptoms on both sides. Energy or information seems to transfer from one side to the other.

- Each point corresponds to a specific point on the acupressure meridians. Hold each point with a steady pressure for one to three minutes. Apply pressure slowly with the tips or balls of the fingers. It is best to place several fingers over the area of the point. If you feel resistance or tens-ion in the area on which you are applying pressure, you may want to push a little harder. However, if your hand starts to feel tense or tired, lighten the pressure a bit. Make sure your hand is comfortable. The acupressure point may feel somewhat tender. This means that the energy pathway or meridian is blocked.

- Expect the tenderness in the point to go away slowly. You may also have a subjective feeling of energy radiating from this point into the body. Many patients describe this sensation as very pleasant. Don't worry if you don't feel it—not everyone does. The main goal is relief from your symptoms.

- Breathe gently while doing each exercise.

- Massage the points once a day or more, whenever you have symptoms of chronic fatigue.

Acupressure Exercises

Exercise 1: Use for Relief of Fatigue and Tiredness

This exercise helps relieve fatigue and tiredness. It stimulates the entire endocrine system because it involves a powerful point for the pituitary gland. This point also helps relax emotional tension as well as relieve eye strain, headaches, hay fever, ulcer pain, and indigestion.

Sit upright on a chair.

Right hand holds point directly between the eyebrows, where the bridge of the nose meets the forehead.

Hold the point for 1 to 3 minutes.

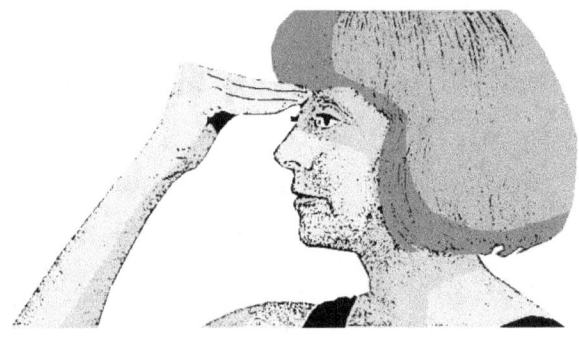

Exercise 2: Use for Relief of Fatigue, Depression, and Immune Dysfunction

This important sequence of points helps relieve upper body tension. The neck and shoulders generally carry a great deal of tension. Tightness in this area can act as a bottleneck and impede the energy flow of the entire body, thus releasing the tightness, energizing the entire body, and relieving fatigue. It also relieves depression and nervous tension. The points in this sequence also strengthen the immune system. A major treatment point for hypoglycemia is worked on in this exercise.

Sit comfortably or lie down. Hold each step for 1 to 3 minutes.

Left hand holds point at the top of the left shoulder blade, 1 to 2 inches to the side of the spine. The point is between the shoulder blade and the spine. It may feel firm and resistant.

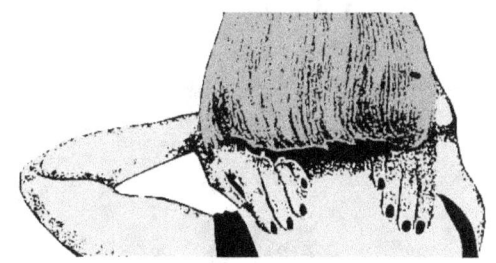

Right hand holds the same point on the right side.

Left hand holds point slightly to the back of the top of the left shoulder where the neck meets the left shoulder.

Right hand holds the same point on the right side.

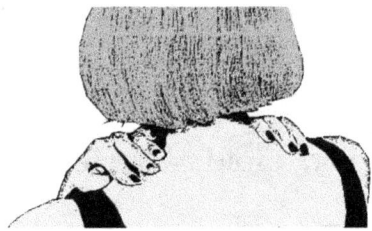

Left hand holds the point halfway up the left side of the neck. Fingers sit on the muscle next to the spine.

Right hand holds the same point on the right side.

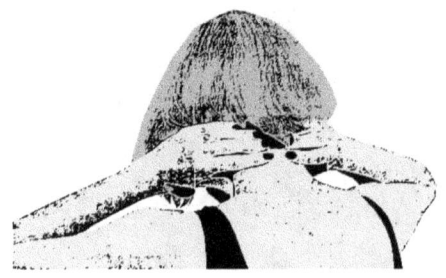

Left hand holds the point at the base of the skull, 1 to 2 inches out from the spine.

Right hand holds the same point on the right side.

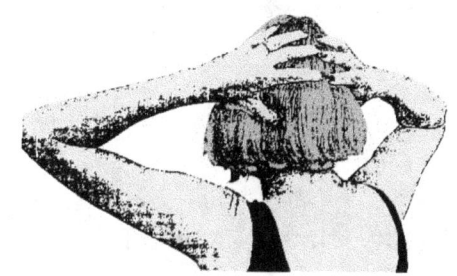

Exercise 3: Use for Relief of Fatigue and Tiredness

This exercise stimulates one of the most important acupressure points for energy, physical stamina, and power. The point stimulated in this exercise, termed the hara in Traditional Chinese Medicine, is considered to be the body's center of gravity. This point also fortifies the digestive tract and helps to strengthen the reproductive system.

Stand or sit upright on a chair.

Fingers hold point below navel. Measure three finger-widths below navel to find this point. The point is located 1 to 2 inches deep inside the abdomen.

Hold the point for 1 to 3 minutes.

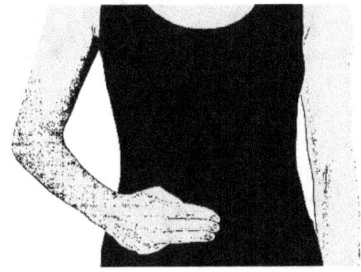

Exercise 4: Use for Relief of Fatigue and Tiredness

This powerful energy point is one of the most important in Chinese medicine. It is used to quickly diminish fatigue and improve energy and endurance. Athletes have traditionally used it to tone and strengthen the muscles as well as increase stamina.

Sit upright on a chair.

Left hand holds point below right knee. This point is located four finger-widths below the kneecap toward the outside of the shinbone. It is sensitive to the touch in many people.

Hold the point for 1 to 3 minutes.

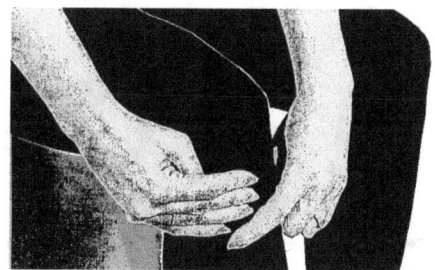

Exercise 5: Improves Immune Function

This sequence of points strengthens the immune system and improves resistance to infections as well as relieving fatigue. This exercise also helps to prevent as well as relieve allergies. It balances the emotions and relieves symptoms of depression.

Sit comfortably or lie down. Hold each step for 1 to 3 minutes.

Left hand holds point on right hand on the webbing between the index finger and thumb. Left thumb is placed on top of the webbing and the index finger is placed underneath the palm. The webbing is squeezed between the thumb and index finger.

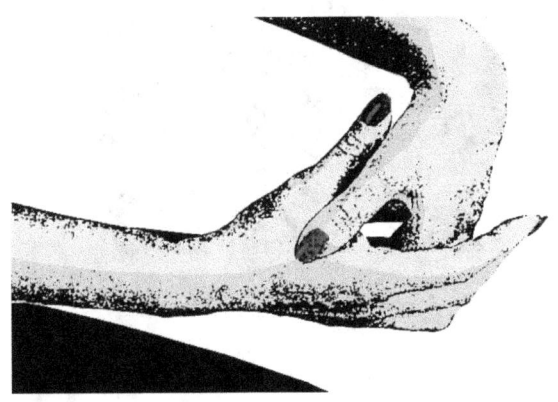

Left hand rubs firmly the area between the bones at the top of the left foot below where the big toe and second toe meet.

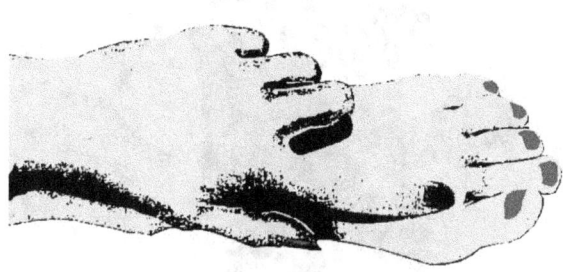

Left and right hands hold points one-half inch below the base of the skull. Fingers will press on the ropy muscles on either side of the spine.

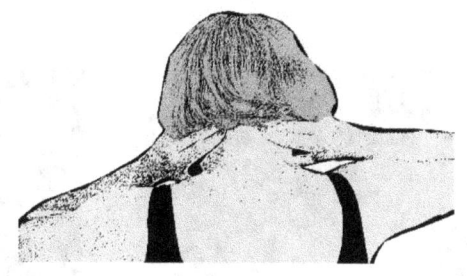

Left hand holds point two finger-widths below the navel.

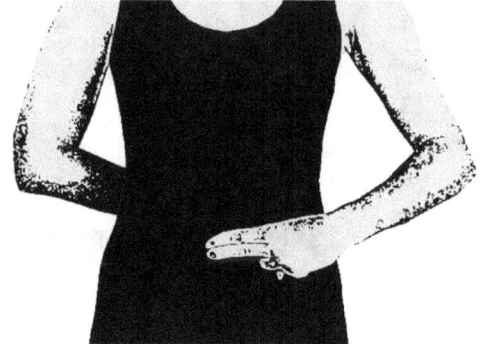

Left hand holds point below right knee. This point is located four finger-widths below the kneecap toward the outside of the shinbone. It is sensitive to the touch in many people.

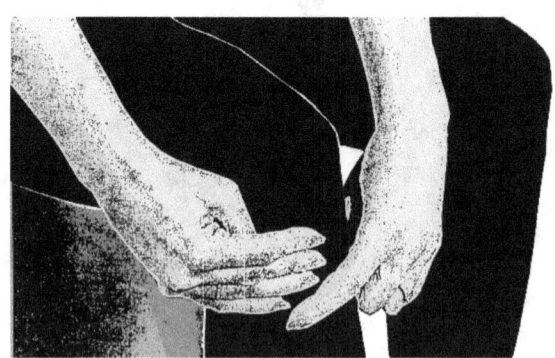

Exercise 6: Relieves Premenstrual and Menopausal Fatigue

This sequence of points relieves the fatigue that women experience prior to the onset of their menstrual periods. For many women with PMS, fatigue is a significant problem that recurs every month. This exercise can also help to relieve menstrual anxiety and depression, as well as menopause-related fatigue. The second step in this sequence has traditionally been forbidden for use by pregnant women after their first trimester.

Sit up and prop your back against a chair. Hold each step 1 to 3 minutes.

Right hand holds point at the base of the ball of the right foot. This point is located between the two pads of the foot.

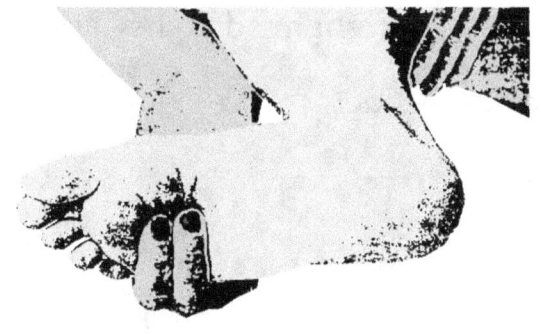

Left hand holds the point midway between the inside of the right anklebone and the Achilles tendon. The Achilles tendon is located at the back of the ankle.

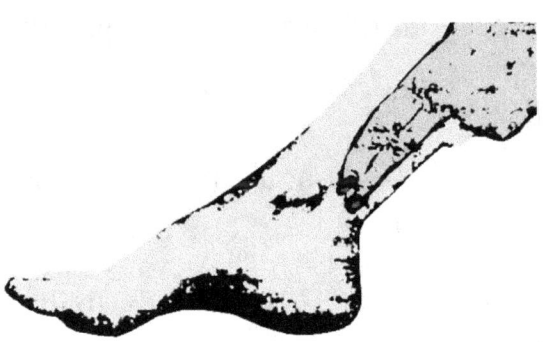

Left hand holds point on right hand at the base of fourth finger.

Repeat sequence on left side.

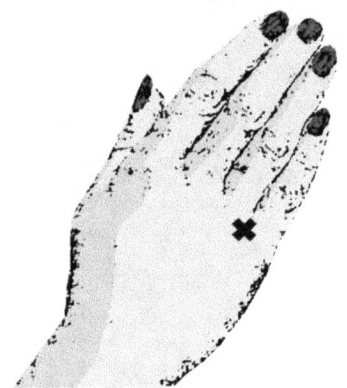

Exercise 7: Use for Relief of Thyroid Imbalance

This exercise energizes the thyroid, whose dysfunction can cause chronic fatigue and tiredness as well as excessive menstrual bleeding, anemia, constipation, and cold intolerance.

Sit upright on a chair. Hold each step for 1 to 3 minutes.

Wrap hands around shoulders with thumbs pressing gently into both sides on top of collarbone.

Fingers are in back. Press against upper shoulders and shoulder blade area.

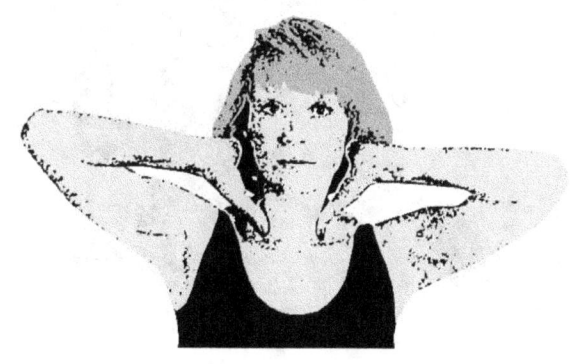

Exercise 8: Use for Relief of Thyroid Imbalance

This exercise helps relieve chronic fatigue and tiredness due to thyroid imbalance. It is used to help stimulate the normal output of thyroid hormone.

Sit upright on a chair.

Fingers touch three points along the large muscle on each side of the neck.

Hold each point for 1 minute

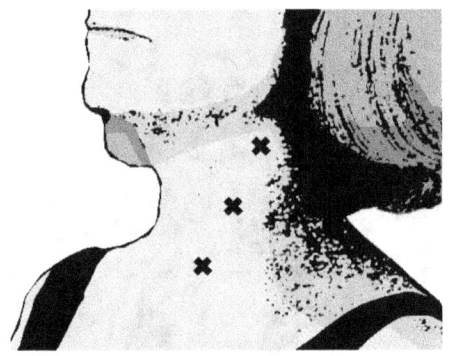

Exercise 9: Use for Relief of Anemia

This sequence of points is important for the treatment of anemia, a common cause of chronic fatigue and tiredness. It involves the stimulation of points on the spleen meridian, related to blood formation and menstrual problems.

Sit upright on a chair. Hold each step for 1 to 3 minutes.

Right hand holds a point four finger widths above the ankle bone.

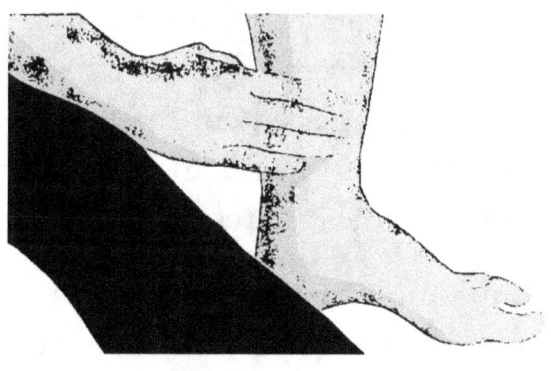

Left hand holds a point over the big toe

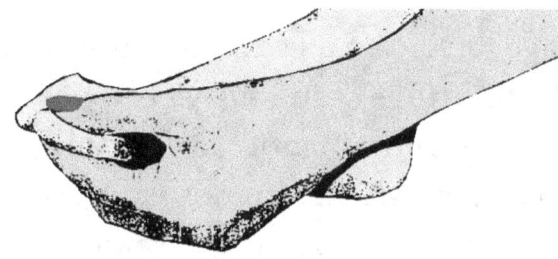

16

Treating Chronic Fatigue with Drugs

Though this book has emphasized the importance and effectiveness of self-care techniques for the treatment of chronic fatigue, medication also has a proper place in certain circumstances. Some cases of chronic fatigue do have treatable causes and these should be properly treated.

As I described in the chapter on diagnosing chronic fatigue, it is important that you have your symptoms evaluated medically by a physician so that any underlying causes needing medication can be treated. If your physician does prescribe medication, monitor its use carefully to avoid negative side effects. However, even in cases where medication may be important—such as hormonal replacement for low thyroid conditions or bioidentical HRT for menopause—I find that combining the medication with self-help techniques gives the best results.

In this chapter, I describe the common drug therapies used for various causes of chronic fatigue. I focus particularly on treatments designed to alleviate fatigue symptoms. Ask your physician for more information about therapies that seem pertinent to your case.

I am going to begin by describing some of the guidelines that I have followed with my own patients in approaching the use of medication for health conditions that may be contributing to your chronic fatigue. You may find these guidelines helpful in dealing with your own situation.

Drugs as Appropriate Therapy

In my own medical practice, I have tended to use drugs as a second line of treatment. I approach the use of drugs cautiously because of their powerful chemical effects on the body and potential for causing toxic side effects and addiction to the medication. My preference is to use the safer and gentler natural therapies such as diet, supplemental nutrients, stress-reduction techniques, deep breathing exercises, counseling, and physical exercises as my first line of treatment whenever possible. Whether you choose to use medication or not, your best long-term results will come from practicing these self-care therapies since they will help to restore your energy and vitality by supporting the health and wellness of your body.

Using Drugs Safely and Effectively

When using drugs for the treatment of chronic fatigue, I always try to prescribe medication only for short-term use and at the lowest therapeutic dose. Unfortunately, drug addiction and unpleasant side effects are real possibilities with the long-term use of certain fatigue reducing drugs, such as antidepressant medication, particularly at high doses. The judicious and careful use of these medications reduces the risk of unpleasant side effects, as well as the withdrawal symptoms that can occur when drugs are discontinued.

Before embarking on a medication program, make sure you understand both the risks and benefits of the medications that you are considering. Discuss with your physician the possible side effects and contraindications to normal activities when using these drugs.

For example, if a drug causes possible sedative effects, you should not attempt to drive a car when these side effects are pronounced. Find out how long your physician plans to keep you on medication and after what time period it will be discontinued to avoid withdrawal effects. Your physician should have a good plan in mind when beginning a program that includes medication.

Good Communication with Your Doctor is Essential

I have always been aware of how important good communication is with my own patients in order to create the best treatment results. I always strive to provide an environment in which my patients feel safe and comfortable in discussing any concerns or issues with me.

It is important that my patients feel that they can ask me any questions or discuss any concerns that they might have. To support this process, I have always set aside plenty of time to talk with my patients during their sessions so that they don't feel that I am rushing to get to the next patient. I want my patients to feel that we are working together as a team and that they can count on me as a strong support system in their lives. This is the kind of medical care that I would want if I were a patient!

Medication always needs to be prescribed by your physician or psychiatrist. If you decide to go on medication, it is important to work with a doctor that you trust and feel comfortable talking about your issues and concerns with. Good communication is important if you are to have the best response to a medication and avoid the pitfall and side-effects that often go along with drug treatments.

To ensure that you have a positive experience with your own physician or caregiver, it is important to share certain information with him or her. For example, before you start on anti-fatigue medication, provide any information to your physician that could affect the use of a particular drug. Pertinent information includes data about any allergies or unusual reactions that you might have to drugs or any other substances, such as foods, preservatives, or dyes. You might also need to use medication for a particular, unrelated, health condition.

Be sure to notify your physician if you are currently taking any other prescription or over-the-counter medications. This will help prevent potentially dangerous drug interactions. Inform your physician if you are pregnant or breastfeeding, because the use of medications can be dangerous to the fetus or nursing infant. If you develop any new medical problem while you are using any of the prescription drugs that I discuss in this chapter, inform your physician immediately.

If you find communication with your physician difficult or you feel uncomfortable talking about your concerns, I suggest that you find another physician with whom you do feel comfortable. The decision about whether to use a particular medication requires a mutual decision on the part of the patient and physician, exchanging full information about the patient's condition and the risks and benefits of the drug. Such matters can be best discussed in a positive patient-doctor relationship.

In the following section of this chapter, I discuss the drugs used most commonly for both the emotional and physical causes of chronic fatigue and tiredness. This should provide you with useful information when making a decision with your physician about drug therapy.

Chronic Fatigue Syndrome/ Myalgic Encephalomyelitis (ME/CFS)

While there are no drugs that cure ME/CFS, a variety of medications have been used by physicians with varying success to try to relieve the symptoms of this condition. These can include:

Antidepressant Medication. Many physicians treat ME/CFS by focusing on symptom relief with antidepressant medication with varying degrees of success. This is done because chronic fatigue often coexists with depression in many women. When given in low dosages, some of the antidepressant medications also improve sleep and reduce pain symptoms.

One tricyclic antidepressant medication, Doxepin has been used to help relieve ME/CFS symptoms. It is a tricyclic antidepressant that may act as an immunomodulator. It has been used to relieve insomnia and induce deep, restful sleep in ME/CFS sufferers. An added benefit for some people with ME/CFS is the ability of doxepin to relieve muscle tension and tightness; it thus acts as a pain-relieving agent. Doxepin can also help relieve general fatigue, nasal congestion, gastritis, and neurological symptoms in ME/CFS sufferers. Side effects include dry mouth, constipation, and weight gain. Other tricyclic antidepressants, such as Sinequan (doxepin hydrochloride) and Elavil (amitriptyline hydrochloride) are also used in ME/CFS therapy.

For more detailed information on these medications, please refer to the previous section.

Non-Steroidal Anti-Inflammatory Drugs (NSAIDs). NSAIDs are sometimes recommended by physicians for the relief of pain and fever that can be associated with ME/CFS. These medications suppress the production of prostaglandins, hormone-like chemicals that can cause pain and cramping. They can also reduce symptoms of fever.

One of the most commonly used NSAIDs is ibuprofen. This drug is sold over the counter as Advil, Motrin or Nuprin, in 200 or 400 milligram dosages, taken every six hours. Ibuprofen should be taken with food as it can cause gastrointestinal upset.

These medications are also available by prescription when taken in higher dosages. They include Motrin (in an 800 milligram dosage), Naprosyn or naproxen sodium as well as Ponstel. These drugs must be used carefully, however, since they can cause gastrointestinal bleeding and peptic ulcer disease or even reactivate a pre-existing ulcer.

Approximately 10 percent of women who use these medications report digestive symptoms, including heartburn, nausea, vomiting, diarrhea, constipation, and poor digestion. To lessen the likelihood of these side effects, always take these medications with food. Report any significant digestive symptoms to your physician. Some women report other unpleasant symptoms when using prostaglandin inhibitors—drowsiness, headaches, vertigo, dizziness, rashes, blurred vision, anemia, edema, and heart palpitations. These drugs can also cause kidney damage. Avoid using these drugs with aspirin, since both can cause gastrointestinal bleeding and irritation.

Valcyte (valganciclovir). Most doctors don't routinely prescribe antimicrobial medication for patients with ME/CFS because researchers haven't identified a particular infectious agent that can be linked to this condition. However, the antiviral drug, Valcyte, has been used in several preliminary small studies to treat patients with documented EBV/ HHV-6 infection that can be found in some patients with ME/CFS.

Human herpesvirus 6 (HHV-6) is a set of herpes viruses that occurs in two related variants: HHV-6A and HHV-6B. These viruses infect nearly all human beings. They often live latent within the body for years, however, can become reactivated later in life.

While small studies have been encouraging, experts in this field agree that larger and better designed studies are needed before they can draw conclusions as to the advisability of recommending this medication in patients with ME/CFS.

H2 Blockers. These are drugs that block the production of stomach acid for the treatment of hiatus hernia, heartburn, and peptic ulcers have been used successfully to treat chronic fatigue patients. These drugs include such commonly used agents as Tagamet (cimetidine hydrochloride) and Zantac (ranitidine hydrochloride). Besides benefiting digestive function, these drugs also act as T-cell immune stimulants and block histamine receptors in T-cells. (Histamine is a chemical that can contribute to nasal congestion, itching, excessive stomach acid, and diarrhea.) These medications may also improve energy, vitality, and alertness in some women with ME/CFS.

Gamma Globulin. This was one of the early medications used to treat ME/CFS, although it is not a commonly used treatment. It provides passive immunity for people suffering from ME/CFS through the injection of a blood product that contains antibodies. ME/CFS sufferers tend to have low levels of IgG subclass I, which normally contains most of our antibodies effective against viruses. Gamma globulin therapy provides these particular antibodies, as well as a whole range of antibodies effective against many viruses, bacteria, and candida.

Gamma globulin is usually given in the intravenous form and is a very expensive form of treatment. Side effects of this treatment include nausea, dizziness, transient flu-like symptoms, headache, and low blood pressure. Another biological drug, Rituxan (rituximab) was found to be useful in treating patients with ME/CFS by researchers in Norway. This drug works by depleting immune cells called B-cells in patients with non-Hodgkins lymphoma, chronic lymphocytic leukemia and rheumatoid arthritis. While symptom relief in most patients was transient, they reported that several patients treated with this drug became symptom-free for several years and were able to return to work.

Depression

Antidepressants are the medications most commonly used to treat depression as well as depression coexisting with anxiety. They are also often prescribed for women with PMS and menopause who suffer from mood symptoms. There are several different types of antidepressant medications that are commonly used in clinical practice today that I discuss in this section.

Selective Serotonin Reuptake Inhibitors (SSRIs). The most commonly prescribed drugs today for the treatment of anxiety as well as depression are the selective serotonin reuptake inhibitors (SSRIs). These medications work by blocking a receptor in the brain that reabsorbs serotonin. This helps to change the balance of serotonin, thereby supporting brain cells to send and receive chemical messages. The end result is an improvement in mood and behavior in women with depression in general and PMS-related depression. Commonly prescribed SSRI's include Prozac (fluoxetine), Celexa (citalopram), Zoloft (sertraline) and Paxil (paroxetine).

The main drawback with these medications is that they are slow to be effective. To begin to feel symptom relief may take between two to eight weeks, so you may not feel better when you initially begin to take these medications. It is important, however, to keep taking them since they are likely to be beneficial once their therapeutic effects start to manifest.

Unlike other mood altering drugs, SSRIs antidepressants are not physically addictive, so the threat of developing withdrawal symptoms is not an issue. However, some women become psychologically addicted to the antidepressants and may have a difficult time weaning themselves off medication. Other side effects include nausea, dry mouth, nervousness, agitation, headache, diarrhea, reduced sexual desire, insomnia and weight gain.

Women who have been taking these medications for a period of time may find that they develop withdrawal symptoms if these medications are abruptly discontinued. They should be gradually tapered off so that the brain can readjust to lower levels of these drugs

Once antidepressants are stopped, the symptoms may recur. Recurrence rate runs between 25 and 50 percent although it can be higher for some women, especially if you've had two or more episodes of depression. The use of these medications for at least six months may also help prevent the recurrence of depression for a longer period of time.

Serotonin and Norepinephrine Reuptake Inhibitors (SNRIs). These medications block the absorption or reuptake and thereby increase your levels of both the inhibitory and excitatory neurotransmitters serotonin and norepinephrine. For some women, these drugs can be more effective in alleviating depression than the use of SSRIs alone. Medications in this group are also called dual-action antidepressants.

Medications of this type include Cymbalta (duloxetine), Effexor XR (venlafaxine) and Pristiq (desvenlafaxine). Side-effects of these medications are usually mild and go away within a few weeks. They include increased sweating, dry mouth, nausea, tiredness, constipation, insomnia and reduced sexual desire.

Norepinephrine and Dopamine Reuptake Inhibitors (NDRIs). NDRIs work by preventing the reuptake of the excitatory neurotransmitters, norepinephrine and dopamine, in the brain. These medications include Wellbutrin (bupropion). Wellbutrin is one of the few antidepressants that doesn't cause diminished sex drive or libido and also helps to suppress appetite and the urge to smoke. However, at high doses it may increase your risk of having seizures. Other side-effects of NDRIs include weight loss, dry mouth, shakiness, headaches, constipation, insomnia and sore throat

Tricyclic Antidepressants. Tricyclic antidepressants, commonly known as "mood elevators," are an older class of antidepressants that are still commonly used today. They produce both an antidepressant and mild tranquilizing effect. Because it takes some time to build up to a therapeutic effect once treatment is initiated, there is a dangerous period of time before the drug takes hold when the patient may remain depressed and become suicidal. However, after two to three weeks of treatment, 80 percent of depressed and anxious patients notice an elevation of mood, increased alertness, and improvement in appetite.

Common tricyclic medications include Elavil (amitriptyline), Tofranil (imipramine), Aventyl (nortriptyline), Norpramin (desipramine) and Sinequan (doxepin). While the actual mechanism of action is not known, it is thought that depression is relieved by elevating the neurotransmitters levels like serotonin and norepinephrine. These are chemicals present in the brain that regulate mood, personality, sleep, and appetite. Many women with depression may lack adequate levels of these neuro-transmitters.

Which of these antidepressants are best suited for depression varies from person to person. The efficiency of any antidepressant depends on each individual's body chemistry. As a result, the patient may have to try several antidepressants to find the one that produces the best therapeutic effect.

Side effects of these drugs are fairly common. In fact, as many as one-quarter of all patients stop therapy with these drugs because of the unpleasant side effects. Many women using antidepressants will initially complain of dry mouth, blurred vision, constipation, drowsiness, weight gain, fatigue, headaches, nausea and even rarely seizures. These symptoms tend to fade in intensity after the first few weeks of taking the medication.

In summary, tricyclic antidepressants can produce much benefit in the short- to intermediate-term treatment of anxiety coexisting with depression, panic episodes, and agoraphobia. They're also useful for the treatment of PMS- and menopause-related depression. However, side effects are common and psychological dependency can develop.

Monoamine oxidase inhibitors (MAOIs). These medications are most likely to be prescribed for women with depression as a last resort, when other medications haven't worked. This is because MAOIs have such significant side effects. Examples of these medications include Parnate (tranylcypromine) and Nardil (phenelzine).

The use of MAOIs requires a strict diet because of dangerous (or even deadly) interactions with foods, such as cheeses, pickles, aged meats and wines as well as avoidance of certain medications including decongestants and cough syrups. Other side effects include dry mouth, nausea, diarrhea, constipation, insomnia, drowsiness, high blood pressure, weight gain, prickling sensation in the skin and reduced sexual desire or difficulty achieving orgasm. A newer MAOI, Emsam (selegiline) can be used as a skin patch rather than taken by mouth. It is thought to cause fewer side effects than other MAOIs. These medications can't be combined with SSRIs.

Fibromyalgia

Non-Steroidal Anti-Inflammatory Drugs (NSAIDs). Many women with fibromyalgia use over-the-counter pain medications for the relief of discomfort. Sometimes, these drugs are effective for pain relief, but they are not effective for everyone. Research studies have found that these drugs provide mild relief of pain, especially when used in combination with mood altering drugs like alprazolam and amitriptyline.

Ibuprofen is often used for fibromyalgia pain relief. This drug is sold over-the-counter as Advil, Motrin or Nuprin, in 200 or 400 milligram dosages. The dose commonly used for menstrual pain and cramps is two tablets, or 400 milligrams, taken every six hours. Like aspirin, ibuprofen should be taken with food as it can cause gastrointestinal upset.

These medications are also available by prescription when taken in higher dosages. They include Motrin (in an 800 milligram dosage), Naprosyn or naproxen sodium as well as Ponstel. These drugs must be used carefully, however, since they can cause gastrointestinal bleeding and peptic ulcer disease or even reactivate a pre-existing ulcer.

Approximately 10 percent of women who use these medications report digestive symptoms, including heartburn, nausea, vomiting, diarrhea, constipation, and poor digestion. To lessen the likelihood of these side effects, always take these medications with food. Report any significant digestive symptoms to your physician. Some women report other unpleasant symptoms when using NSAIDs—drowsiness, headaches, vertigo, dizziness, rashes, blurred vision, anemia, edema, and heart palpitations. Avoid using these drugs with aspirin, since both can cause gastrointestinal bleeding and irritation.

Other Pain Relievers. Some physicians also prescribe tramadol (Ultram), which is often used to treat fibromyalgia pain. Tramadol is a narcotic-like pain reliever used to treat moderate to severe pain. Several research studies support its benefit in relieving pain in conditions such as fibromyalgia, low back pain and osteoarthritis.

There are certain drawbacks to using this medication, particularly its risk of becoming habit-forming and causing an addiction in the user. It also has been known to cause side-effects such as abdominal or stomach pain, constipation or diarrhea, headache, drowsiness, cough, agitation, anxiety, nasal congestion, muscle aches and pains, difficulty concentrating, sweating, skin rash and even seizures in some people. Tramadol should not be used if you are taking narcotic pain medication, sedatives, tranquilizers or antidepressant or antianxiety medication.

Antidepressant Medication. Tricyclic antidepressants have been found to be effective for the treatment of fibromyalgia, headaches related to chronic tension and pain related to muscle spasm. They are also useful for treating the sleep disturbances that are very common in women with fibromyalgia. Sleep disturbances are often treated successfully with low doses of tricyclic antidepressants, such as Elavil (amitriptyline), Sinequan (doxepin) and Pamelor and Aventyl (nortriptyline). Sometimes doctors may prescribe sleeping pills for short-term use.

Women with fibromyalgia may also experience depression and other mood-related issues. The symptoms of depression can be treated with selective serotonin reuptake inhibitors (SSRIs) such as (fluoxetine) Prozac and Zoloft (sertraline). They have also been effective for relieving fibromyalgia-related pain, sleep deprivation and improving an overall sense of well-being in these patients.

The main drawback with these medications is that they are slow to be effective. To begin to feel symptom relief may take between two to eight weeks, so you may not feel better when you initially begin to take these medications. It is important, however, to keep taking them since they are likely to be beneficial once their therapeutic effects start to manifest.

Muscle Relaxants. Low doses of the muscle relaxant Flexeril (cyclobenaza-prine) have been shown to have some therapeutic benefits for fibromyalgia patients, according to a small study published in *The Journal of Rheumatology*.

When taken at bedtime, cyclobenazaprine was helpful in promoting more restful sleep with total sleep time increasing from an average of 5.7 hours to 6.4 hours. Pain declined by 26 percent and tenderness decreased by 30 percent in the group of patients taking the drug. In addition, depression declined by 22 percent in the patients receiving the drug. Headaches were the most common side effect reported by the patients along with dry mouth and drowsiness.

Muscle relaxants should not, however, be prescribed at higher doses for fibromyalgia patients since they can cause drowsiness during the daytime hours and make it difficult for patients to function in their everyday lives.

Anticonvulsants. These medications may have some benefit in providing symptom relief for fibromyalgia patients. There is one controlled study of pregabalin that showed reduction of pain, fatigue and sleep disturbance compared to the placebo when taken at a dosage of 450 mg per day. The most common side-effects reported by patients were dizziness and sleepiness.

Another double-blind, placebo controlled study of 150 mostly women patients was done at the Women's Health Research Program at the University of Cincinnati College of Medicine. In this study, researchers found that patients taking gabapentin at dosages of 1,200 to 2,400 mg daily for 12 weeks had significantly less pain than those taking the placebo. The patients taking gabapentin also reported much better sleep and less fatigue. For the majority of participants, the drug was well tolerated. The most common side effects included dizziness and sedation, which were mild to moderate in severity in most cases.

PMS and Depression

PMS-related depression and fatigue, may be relieved by antidepressants. Antidepressant medications may help to correct the chemical basis of the underlying depression and often bring positive relief of symptoms within three to eight weeks. These medications should be used cautiously and only if the more gentle self-care treatments fail, because they are very powerful drugs and unfortunately can cause significant side effects. They should be used only when prescribed and supervised by a knowledgeable physician. Antidepressant medications are discussed in detail earlier in this chapter in the section on depression. I recommend that you refer to that section for more detailed information.

Some physicians recommend the use of bioidentical progesterone as a treatment for moderate to severe PMS symptoms. Bioidentical hormones are identical to those produced by our own bodies rather than the types of HRT usually prescribed by conventional physicians. Conventional forms of HRT differ both in their chemical make-up and how they affect your body. Bioidentical progesterone can be taken as a skin cream, gel, sub-lingual tablets, sprays and pills. Though progesterone can be a helpful treatment for PMS anxiety, irritability, and mood swings, women with PMS-related fatigue and depression should use it cautiously. Progesterone has sedative properties, and in high levels can be used as an anesthetic.

If you have specific questions about the appropriateness of progesterone for treatment of your PMS, ask your physician. Some doctors occasionally prescribe birth control pills for PMS in an attempt to reduce symptoms by suppressing ovulation. The progestins or synthetic progesterone in oral contraceptives can worsen fatigue and depression, particularly if the pill is progesterone-dominant.

Women with PMS-related fatigue and depression also need to be careful using some commonly prescribed PMS medications. Diuretics can be helpful in the short term for reducing PMS-related fluid retention and bloating. However, they also deplete the body's store of essential minerals, such as potassium and calcium. Over time, depletion of minerals can worsen chronic fatigue.

Menopause

Many menopausal women find that the use of hormonal replacement therapy (HRT) gives their mood and energy level a tremendous boost. I recommend the use of bioidentical hormones because they are identical to the hormones produced by our own bodies rather than the synthetic or semi-synthetic types of HRT usually prescribed by conventional physicians. Conventional forms of HRT differ both in their chemical make-up and how they affect your body.

Estrogen is usually prescribed as a pill, patch or vaginal cream while progestins are given as a pill. There are many brands on the market, generally composed of combinations of two types of estrogen that occur naturally in your body: estrone and estradiol. Estrone is the main type of estrogen that your body makes after menopause, while estradiol is present in greater amounts during your menstrual years.

Both synthetic and naturally derived estrogen are available. The most popular brand is Premarin (conjugated estrogen tablets), which comes from the urine of pregnant mares and contains a natural mixture of estrogen, including estrone. Other popular brands include Ogen (estropipate tablets), which contains estrone; Estrace (estradiol tablets), which contains estradiol; and many other generic formulations.

Conventional HRT. Let's spend a few minutes and look at the issues surrounding the use of conventional HRT. The issue of whether to use hormones or not is a question that most menopausal women pursue with their own physician as well as with friends and through reading materials. Statistically, estrogen and progestin use is much lower than most women suspect. Only 15 percent of women in the menopause and postmenopause age group actually use hormonal replacement therapy (HRT). The women who choose not to use HRT often do so because their symptoms are mild or absent or they have many concerns about the possible immediate and long-term side effects that could occur with the use of hormones.

This has become a major issue for women in menopause since 2002 after a government commissioned study, the Women's Health Initiative, found that HRT could increase the risk of breast cancer, heart attack, strokes and blood clots. Synthetic forms of progesterone, called progestins like Provera, have traditionally been prescribed for menopausal women.

Unfortunately, progestins can worsen fatigue and depression in susceptible women. This can be a significant issue if you suffer from chronic fatigue. Women with coexisting anxiety and depression should use them cautiously while conventional forms of estrogen therapy can sometimes worsen anxiety. However, while these negative findings have continued to accumulate in studies done since this time, other research trials have found that HRT does have benefits such as the reduction of vaginal pain, dryness and hot flashes.

Bioidentical Hormones. In contrast, bioidentical hormones are much less likely to cause side-effects. Bioidentical estrogen is primarily composed of a much lower potency form of estrogen, called estriol that we also produce within our bodies. Because of its lower potency, estriol causes much less side effects in women.

With the use of bioidentical estrogen and progesterone, many of my patients have reported not only relief from hot flashes and vaginal dryness, but also more energy, mood stabilization, and improved sex drive. Depression, the blues, and fatigue are often eradicated, as are insomnia, irritability, and edginess. They also usually found that they tolerated bioidentical hormones better than conventional HRT, which they may have tried initially. Bioidentical estrogen can be taken either in pill form, patch, skin cream, vaginal cream or as a pellet.

Occasionally, women in menopause may have to resort to the use of antidepressants if their fatigue and depression are not relieved by the use of hormones. Refer to the section on PMS medication for more specific information on common antidepressant medications.

Weak Adrenals

Prednisone. This medication belongs to a class of drug called corticosteroids. It prevents the release of substances in the body that normally would cause inflammation. It also decreases your immune system's response to stress and various diseases. The end result is that prednisone reduces symptoms of inflammation and swelling as healthy, strong adrenal glands would be more likely to do. Prednisone is prescribed by doctors to treat conditions such as severe allergies, rheumatoid arthritis, eczema, psoriasis, lung problems affecting breathing, ulcerative colitis, lupus and other health issues.

Prednisone should be taken by mouth with a meal, usually in the morning and then earlier in the day if you are taking it more than once a day. Taking prednisone at night should be avoided since it can have a stimulant effect and cause sleeplessness or insomnia. Physicians will usually prescribe it in a higher dosage initially, often at the 50 to 60 mg dosage level, to promote a therapeutic effect and then taper the dosage down sharply over a week or two. Although prednisone is often very effective when used for short-term therapy, it should not be used on a long-term basis, longer than a month, since it can cause severe side-effects.

Side effects can include nausea, vomiting, heartburn, insomnia, increased sweating or acne. Other side effects are muscle pain or cramping, unusual weight gain, bloody or tarry bowel movements, blurred vision, irregular heartbeat, depression or agitation. Steroid medication like prednisone can weaken your immune system, making it easier for you to get an infection.

It is important to watch for signs such as fever or persistent sore throat that can indicate an infectious disease. It shouldn't be used at all if you already have a fungal disease anywhere in your body. Long term use of prednisone can cause thinning of the skin, seizures, elevation of the blood sugar level and bone loss. Prednisone shouldn't be used during pregnancy since it can cause low birth weight or birth defects.

Dosages can vary with 60 mg often being prescribed on the high side and 5 mg on the low end as the drug is tapered down. Side effects are more likely to occur at dosages greater than 20 mg per day. There are studies, however, that have shown very low dosages of prednisone can be used for much longer periods of time and provide substantial therapeutic benefits. For example, dosages of prednisone at the 2 mg and 3 mg levels for extended periods of time, up to two years or more, have been found to be very well tolerated by rheumatoid arthritis patients and effective in reducing the progression of the disease in a number of studies.

Hypothyroidism

Another treatable cause of anemia-related fatigue is low thyroid function. Hypothyroidism is easily treatable by thyroid replacement therapy. Besides correcting fatigue and tiredness, thyroid replacement therapy corrects other common symptoms of thyroid deficiency, including constipation, skin and hair changes, weight gain, excessive menstrual bleeding, and elevated blood cholesterol levels.

A thyroid imbalance must be carefully managed by a physician through blood tests and office evaluation so the proper dose can be prescribed. Most people who suffer from thyroid conditions are female (90 percent of the total hypo-thyroid cases in the United States are women), so it is a common condition frequently seen by physicians who specialize in women's health care.

While most conventional physicians prescribe only the predominant thyroid hormone, thyroxine (T4), for replacement therapy, most alternative physicians prefer to use a combination of T4 and T3 (triiodothyronine) because they feel that they have better results regarding the mood-related symptoms that are commonly seen in women with chronic fatigue as well as thyroid disease.

In conclusion, many drug therapies may be helpful in treating either the causes or symptoms of various forms of chronic fatigue. Unfortunately, quite a few of these drugs may have side effects that are quite difficult for women with chronic fatigue to handle. Check with your own physician for specific guidelines on these medications.

Candida Infections

Physicians now commonly treat candida albicans infections with three prescription medications. Nystatin has been prescribed as an oral medication since the late 1970s to eradicate yeast in the intestinal tract. It is available in tablet, capsule, liquid solution, and powder form. Nystatin is used frequently to treat candida-infected patients who complain of fatigue, depression, headaches, and PMS symptoms.

Nizoral (ketoconazole) is an antifungal medication that has been used in the United States since 1981. Nizoral has been used successfully by physicians for yeast infections that are more difficult to eradicate, along with a sugar-free diet (which should be used by all candida-infected patients). The medication may occasionally cause serious side effects. Because of this, liver function should be monitored every few weeks in women taking the medication for one month or more.

Diflucan (fluconazole) is a broad-spectrum antifungal agent related to Nizoral. It is the most recently introduced of the three medications in the United States, although it has had previous use in Europe. It is absorbed into the body through the intestines after oral administration. Studies suggest that it is a more powerful antifungal agent than Nizoral and causes less toxic side effects. Side-effects can include nausea and abdominal discomfort.

Allergies

Antihistamine and decongestant medications are frequently used to control the common symptoms of allergies. Yet one of the main side effects of these medications is sedation. In fact, some women use antihistamines specifically for their side effects—to induce sleep—as an alternative to stronger sleep medication. These drugs should be used cautiously by women with chronic fatigue, especially while working and driving. A better approach is the eradication of allergens through an anti-fatigue, low-stress diet and the elimination of allergens from the physical environment, in order to reduce the dependence on antihistamines and decongestants in an allergic woman with chronic fatigue.

Anemia

In some cases drug therapy can correct anemia, if it addresses the underlying cause of the problem. For instance, hormonal therapy can help correct anemia caused by heavy menstrual bleeding. This problem is often seen in teenagers and in women who are in transition into menopause.

Anemia may become particularly acute in premenopausal women because of hormonal instability. As the ovarian follicles lose the ability to produce estrogen and progesterone, premenopausal women begin to ovulate less frequently. The menstrual cycle often shortens, with periods coming closer together. Bleeding may become heavier and last longer. A menstrual period lasting 7 to 10 days is fairly common. In extreme cases, women may bleed 60 or more consecutive days. As menopause approaches, this instability corrects itself. Periods become farther apart, and the flow becomes lighter until menstruation finally ceases.

It is during this phase of heavy menstrual bleeding that women are most likely to need medical care. Often the bleeding can be stopped by the use of bioidentical progesterone. As previously described, this is identical to the progesterone that you produce within your body. It acts much the way your own natural progesterone does, by limiting the amount of bleeding from the uterine lining during the second half of the menstrual cycle.

Unfortunately, most conventional physicians prescribe a synthetic progesterone-like hormone called a progestin. Provera is the type used most often in the United States; administered orally for one or two weeks, this drug can usually stop the bleeding. It also limits the amount of bleeding from the uterine lining during the second half of the menstrual cycle. Although Provera can be quite effective in stopping heavy menstrual bleeding, it does cause side effects in some women. The most common are depression and fatigue. Therefore, Provera can act as a double-edged sword: correcting fatigue by stopping heavy bleeding and anemia, while worsening fatigue in some women who are already tired and exhausted. I definitely recommend the use of bioidentical progesterone over Provera if you are suffering from chronic fatigue.

17

How to Put Your Program Together

I hope you that have enjoyed my book and found it useful. I have shared with you a complete self-care program to prevent and relieve your symptoms of chronic fatigue and tiredness. My program will help to restore your energy, vitality and stamina and eliminate any stressors that have been depleting and exhausting your body. It will also support the health of essential systems including your brain and nervous systems, hormones and digestive function and immunity necessary for a high level of energy. Your general health and well-being should benefit greatly from this program.

I have shared many helpful and effective treatment options with you. Try the therapies that appeal to you the most. I recommend that you make them part of your daily routine so that you can receive the most benefit from them.

I usually recommend beginning any self-care program slowly so you can comfortably become accustomed to the lifestyle changes. People differ in their ability to adjust to major lifestyle changes. Though some of my patients like to eliminate their old, unhealthy habits as quickly as possible, other women find such rapid changes in their long-term habits to be too stressful. Find the pace that works for you.

Enjoy the program. I always tell my patients to regard their self-care program as an enjoyable adventure. The menus and food selections I've recommended in this book provide you with an opportunity to try delicious and healthful new recipes and meal plans. The stretching exercises, acupressure points and stress-reduction exercises have also been developed to help support your health and vitality.

As you do the program, don't set up unrealistic or overly strict expectations for yourself. You don't have to be perfect to get great results.

Healing is a cumulative process and all of the positive changes that you make will be beneficial. Follow the guidelines of the program as well as you can and as your schedule permits.

It is not a major issue if you occasionally forget to take your vitamins or don't have time to exercise on a particular day. Don't be discouraged if you can't follow the dietary recommendations on vacations, holidays, and birthdays. Periodically review the guidelines outlined in this book and continue to adapt your lifestyle to the healthful suggestions that I've shared with you. Over time you will notice many beneficial changes.

Be your own feedback system. Your body will tell you if you are on the right track and if what you are doing is making you feel better. It will also tell you if your current diet and emotional stresses are making your symptoms worse. Remember that even moderate changes in your habits can make significant differences.

The Chronic Fatigue Workbook

Fill out the workbook section of this book. The questionnaires will help you determine which areas in your life have contributed the most to your fatigue symptoms and need the most improvement. Then, by reviewing the workbook every month or two as you follow the self-help program, you will see the areas in which you are making the most progress, with both symptom relief and initiation of healthier lifestyle habits. The workbook can provide feedback in an organized and easy-to-use manner.

Diet and Nutritional Supplements

I recommend that you make all nutritional changes gradually. It is important to eliminate foods that may be contributing to your fatigue and tiredness and add foods that support your energy and emotional and physical health. Many women find breakfast the easiest meal to change because it is simple and often eaten at home. To change your other meals and snacks, periodically review the lists of foods to eliminate and those to emphasize.

Each month, pick a few foods that you are willing to eliminate from your diet. Try in their place the foods that help prevent and relieve chronic fatigue. The recipes and menus that I have shared with you should be very helpful. Use the meal plans as helpful guidelines while you restructure your diet to suit your needs.

Vitamins, minerals, essential fatty acids, amino acids and herbal supplements will help complete your nutritional program and speed up the healing process. Most women find the nutritional supplement program to be a very important part of their chronic fatigue program. The use of nutritional supplements can help greatly to promote a calm and relaxed mood.

Stress Reduction and Breathing Exercises

The stress-reduction and breathing exercises can play an important role in supporting your emotional and physical healing process. I also suggest trying the light, water, and sound therapies for added benefit. I find that all my patients heal more rapidly and find that they have more energy when they are calm, happy, and relaxed.

These exercises have been designed to induce a state of energy and vitality along with a feeling of deep peace and calm. They will also help to reinforce new ways of handling stress. When practiced on a regular basis, they help build confidence in your ability to handle any issues that may have been depleting you. The visualization and affirmation exercises can help you create a blueprint in your mind for optimal emotional health and well-being. This will enable your body and mind to work together in greater harmony.

Begin by trying the stress-reduction and breathing exercises that most appeal to you. Choose the combination that works best for you. Practice stress management on a regular basis and be aware of your habitual breathing patterns. Both of these techniques will help you relax and release the tensions that worsen your fatigue. They will help induce a sense of peace and well-being. They will also help to repattern your nervous system and brain chemistry so that you are able to handle stress better and feel much more peaceful and calm on a consistent basis.

You do not need to spend enormous amounts of time on these exercises. Even 10 minutes out of your daily schedule can be helpful. You may find that the quietest times for you are early in the morning before you get out of bed or late at night before going to sleep.

You might also choose to take a "breath break" or meditation break during the day. You can close the door to your office or go into your bedroom at home for 10 minutes to relax. Use the time to breathe deeply, do the visualizations, or meditate. You will be much calmer and more relaxed afterward and it will help to boost your energy.

Physical Exercise

Women with chronic fatigue should do moderate exercise on a regular basis, at least three times a week. Aerobic exercise, such as walking, is tremendously useful in treating fatigue since it improves oxygenation and blood circulation to your brain and the rest of your body. This will help to restore your health and well-being.

Begin slowly, even exercising for just a few minutes a day will be very beneficial in helping to build your energy. Aerobic exercise, such as walking, is tremendously useful in treating fatigue since it improves oxygenation and blood circulation to your brain and the rest of your body. This will help to restore your health and well-being.

If you are very tired, just take a walk around the block where you live and then start to slowly increase the distance. If you do this regularly, you will find that as your stamina improves, you will be able to walk longer and longer distances. It is important to do your exercise routine in a slow, comfortable manner, so as not to worsen your symptoms. Frenetic exercise that is too fast-paced is unhealthy if you are already fatigued since it can actually exhaust you further. Pick a tempo that feels relaxing and comfortable.

If you are interested in doing the stretches and acupressure massage points described in this book, I recommend that you set aside fifteen minutes to half-hour each day for the first week or two of starting your self-help program. Try the exercises that appeal to you and offer correction for your specific set of symptoms. After an initial period of exploration, choose the ones that you enjoy the most and that seem to give you the most relief. Practice them on a regular basis so they can help prevent and reduce your symptoms.

Conclusion

I want to inspire you that you have a tremendous ability to heal and that you can enjoy greater energy as well as radiant health and well-being. By working with the very effective treatment programs contained in this book, you can create more energy, vitality and stamina along with more peace and relaxation in your life. You will also find that you begin to have a greatly improved ability to handle the day-to-day stresses of your life. Practicing healthy nutritional habits, exercising daily or every other day and doing the relaxation and stress-reduction techniques will provide you with great benefits.

By combining these beneficial principles of self-care, you can enjoy the same wonderful results that my patients have had in banishing chronic fatigue from their lives and enjoying each day with a renewed sense of energy and vitality.

To your great health!

Love,

Dr. Susan

About Susan Richards M.D.

Dr. Susan Richards is one of the foremost authorities in the fields of family medicine and alternative medicine. Dr. Richards has successfully treated many thousands of patients emphasizing alternative health and integrative medicine in her clinical practice. Her mission is to provide her patients with safe and effective alternative therapies to greatly enhance their health and well-being.

A graduate of Northwestern University Feinberg School of Medicine, she has served on the clinical faculty of Stanford University School of Medicine and taught in their Division of Family and Community Medicine.

Her Facebook page, Dr. Susan's Healthy Living, has over one million followers. She is also an ordained minister and her ministry receives over a million prayer requests for healing each year.

Notes

Notes

Notes

References

"Does Vitamin B12 Help Relieve Fatigue?"
(http://www.medscape.com/viewarticle/585589). Medscape.
http://www.medscape.com/viewarticle/585589. Retrieved 2010-12-10.

A Behan PO, Behan WM, Horrobin D (1990). "Effect of high doses of essential fatty acids on the postviral fatigue syndrome". *Acta Neurol. Scand.* **82** (3): 209-16. doi:10.1110.1600-0404.199011304490.x (http://dx.doi.org/10.1111%2Fj.1600-0404.1990.tb04490.x) . PMID 2270749 (http://www.ncbi.nlm.nih.gov/pubmed/2270749).

A Kreijkamp-Kaspers S, Brenu EW, Marshall S, Staines D, Van Driel ML. (November 2011). "Treating chronic fatigue syndrome - a study into the scientific evidence for pharmacological treatments." (http://www.racgp.org.au/afp/201111/201111kkaspers.pdf). *Aust Fam Physician* **40 (11):** 907-12. PMID 22059223 (http://www.ncbi.nlm.nih.gov/pubmed/22059223). http://www.racgp.org.au/afp/201111/201111kkaspers.pdf.

A Luyten P, Van Houdenhove B, Pae CU, Kempke S, Van Wambeke P (December 2008). "Treatment of chronic fatigue syndrome: findings, principles and strategies." (http://www.ncbi.nlm.nih.gov/pmc/articles/PMC2796012) . *Psychiatry Investig* 5 (4): 209-12. PMID 20046339 (http://www.ncbi.nlm.nih.gov/pubmed/20046339) . http://www.ncbi.nlm.nih.gov/pmc/articles/PMC2796012.

Afari N, Eisenberg DM, Herrell R et al. (2000). "Use of alternative treatments by chronic fatigue syndrome discordant twins". *Integr Med* **2** (2): 97-103. doi:10.1016/S1096-2190(99)00017-7 (http://dx.doi.org/10.1016%2FS1096 2190%2899%2900017-7) . PMID 10882883 (http://www.ncbi.nlm.nih.gov/pubmed/10882883).

Armanini D, Lewicka S, Pratesi C, et al. Further studies on the mechanism of the mineralocorticoid action of licorice in humans. J Endocrinol Invest 1996;19:624-9.

Avellaneda Fernandez A, Perez Martin A, Izquierdo Martinez M, et al. Chronic fatigue syndrome: aetiology, diagnosis and treatment. BMC Psychiatry 2009;9 Suppl 1:S1.

Bates DW, Buchwald D, Lee J, et al. Clinical laboratory test findings in patients with chronic fatigue syndrome. Arch Intern Med 1995;155:97-103.

Behan PO, Behan WM, Horrobin D. Effect of high doses of essential fatty acids on the postviral fatigue syndrome. *Acta Neurol Scand.* 1990;82:209-216.

Brouwers FM, Van Der Werf S, Bleijenberg G, et al. The effect of a polynutrient supplement on fatigue and physical activity of patients with chronic fatigue syndrome: a double-blind randomized controlled trial. *QJM.* 2002;95:677-683.

CDC ME/CFS Toolkit. Centers for Disease Control and Prevention. September 6, 2011. Available at: http://www.cdc.gov/ME/CFS/toolkit/index.html (Accessed 06 January 2012).

Clague JE, Edwards RH, Jackson MJ. Intravenous magnesium loading in chronic fatigue syndrome. Lancet 1992;340:124-5.

Cleare AJ, Heap E, Malhi GS, et al. Low-dose hydrocortisone in chronic fatigue syndrome: a randomized crossover trial. *Lancet.* 1999;353:455-458.

Consultation letter MLX 286: Proposals to prohibit the herbal ingredient Kava-Kava (Piper methysticum) in unlicensed medicines. Medicines Control Agency, United Kingdom, July 19, 2002.

Cox IM, Campbell MJ, Dowson D (1991). "Red blood cell magnesium and chronic fatigue syndrome". *Lancet* **337** (8744): 757-60. doi:10.1016/0140-6736(91)91371-Z (http://dx.doi.org/10.1016%2F0140-6736%2891%2991371-Z) . PMID 1672392 (http://www.ncbi.nlm.nih.gov/pubmed/1672392).

Cunha BA. Beta-carotene stimulation of natural killer cell activity in adult patients with chronic fatigue syndrome. *CFIDS Chronicle Physicians' Forum.* 1993:18-19.

Deale A, Chalder T, Wessely S. Commentary on randomized, double-blind, placebo-controlled trial of fluoxetine and graded exercise for chronic fatigue syndrome. *BrJ Psychiatry.* 1998;172:491-492.

Deale A, Husain K, Chalder T, Wessely S (December 2001). "Long-term outcome of cognitive behavior therapy versus relaxation therapy for chronic fatigue syndrome: a 5-year follow-up study" (http://ajp.psychiatryonline.org/cgi/pmidlookup?view=long&pmid=11729022).

Am J Psychiatry **158 (12):** 2038-42. doi:10.1176/appi .ajp .158.12.2038 (http://dx.doi .org/10.1176%2Fappi .ajp.158.12.2038) . PMID 11729022

Derek Pheby, Lisa Saffron (Oct-Dec 2009). "Risk factors for severe ME/ME/CFS."

Dessein PH, Shipton EA. Hydrocortisone and chronic fatigue syndrome [letter]. *Lancet.* 1999;353:1618. Baschetti R. Hydrocortisone and chronic fatigue syndrome [letter] *Lancet.* 1999;353:1618.

Deulofeu R, Gascon J, Gimenez N, Corachan M. Magnesium and chronic fatigue syndrome. Lancet 1991;338:641.

Drug Intervention in Chronic Fatigue Syndrome (http://clinicaltrials.gov/ct2/show/NCT00848692?term=chronic+fatigue+syndrome&rank=4)

Durlach J. Chronic fatigue syndrome and chronic primary magnesium deficiency (ME/CFS and CPMD). *Magnes Res.* 1992;5:68.

Edmonds M, McGuire H, Price J (2004). Price, Jonathan R. ed. "Exercise therapy for chronic fatigue syndrome" (http://mrw .interscience.wiley.com/cochrane/clsysrev/articles/CD003200/frame.html). *Cochrane Database Syst Rev* (3): CD003200. doi:10.1002/14651858.CD003200.pub2 (http://dx.doi.org/10.1002%2F14651858.CD003200.pub2).

Escher M, Desmeules J, Giostra E, Mentha G. Hepatitis associated with Kava, a herbal remedy for anxiety. BMJ 2001;322:139.

Gantz NM. Magnesium and chronic fatigue. Lancet 1991;338:66.

Grant JE, Veldee MS, Buchwald D. Analysis of dietary intake and selected nutrient concentrations in patients with chronic fatigue syndrome. J Am Diet Assoc 1996;96:383-6.

Hartz A, Bentler S, Noyes R, et al. Randomized controlled trial of Siberian ginseng for chronic fatigue. *Psycho/ Med.* 2004;34:51-61.

Heath M, Klein NC, Cunha BA. Dose dependent effects of beta carotene therapy in chronic fatigue syndrome [abstract]. *Clin Res.* 1994;42:345A.

Himmel PB, Seligman TM. A Pilot Study Employing Dehydroepiandrosterone (DHEA) in the Treatment of Chronic Fatigue Syndrome. [Abstract]. J Clin Rheumatol 1999:5:56-9.

Hinds G, Bell NP, McMaster D, McCluskey DR. Normal red cell magnesium concentrations and magnesium loading tests in patients with chronic fatigue syndrome. Ann Clin Biochem 1994;31:459-61.

Howard JM, Davies S, Hunnisett A. Magnesium and chronic fatigue syndrome [letter]. *Lancet*. 1992;340A26.

Inazu M, Matsumiya T (June 2008). "[Physiological functions of carnitine and carnitine transporters in the central nervous system]" (in Japanese). *Nihon Shinkei Seishin Yakurigaku Zasshi* **28** (3): 113-20. PMID 18646596 (http://www.ncbi.nlm.nih.gov/pubmed/18646596).

Int J Mol Med 1998;1:143-6.

Jackson JL, O'Malley PG, Kroenke K (March 200). "Antidepressants and cognitive-behavioral therapy for symptom syndromes" (http://www.cnsspectrums.corn/aspx/articledetail.aspx?articleid=417). *CNS Spectr* **11** (3): 212-22.

Jeffcoate WJ. Chronic fatigue syndrome and functional hypoadrenia-fighting vainly the old ennui [letter]. *Lancet*. 1999;353:424-425.

Kaslow JE, Rucker L, Onishi R. Liver extract-folic acid-cyanocobalamin vs placebo for chronic fatigue syndrome. Arch Intern Med 1989;149:2501-3.

Kavelaars A, Kuis W, Knook L, et al. Disturbed neuroendocrine-immune interactions in chronic fatigue syndrome. J Clin Endocrinol Metab 2000;85:692-6.

Knoop H, Bleijenberg G, Gielissen MF, van der Meer JW, White PD (2007). "Is a full recovery possible after cognitive behavioural therapy for chronic fatigue syndrome?". *Psychother Psychosom* **76** (3): 171-6. doi:10.1159/000099844 (http://dx.doi.org/10.1159%2F000099844) . PMID 17426416 (http://www.ncbi.nlm.nih.gov/pubmed/17426416).

Lloyd AR, Hickie I, Brockman A, et al. Immunologic and psychologic therapy for patients with chronic fatigue syndrome: a double-blind, placebo-controlled trial. Am J Med 1993;94:197-203.

Lynch S, Fraser). Fluoxetine and graded exercise in chronic fatigue syndrome [letter]. *BrJ Psychiatry.* 1998;173:353.

Malaguarnera M, Gargante MP, Cristaldi E et al. (2008). "Acetyl L-carnitine (ALC) treatment in elderly patients with fatigue". *Arch Gerontol Geriatr* **46** (2): 181-90. doi:10.1016/j.archger.2007.03.012 (http://dx.doi.org/10.1016%2Fj.archger2007.03.012). PMID 17658628 (http://www.ncbi.nlm.nih.gov/pubmed/17658628).

Malouff JM et al. (June 2008). "Efficacy of cognitive behavioral therapy for chronic fatigue syndrome: a meta-analysis". *Clin Psychol Rev* **28** *(5):* 736-45. doi:10.1016/j.cpr.2007.10.004 (http://dx.doi.org/10.1016%2Fj.cpr.2007.10.004). PMID 18060672 (http://www.ncbi.nlm.nih.gov/pubmed/18060672).

Mark A. Demitrack, Susan E. Abbey (1999). *Chronic Fatigue Syndrome: An Integrative Approach to Evaluation and Treatment.* Guilford Press. pp. 241. ISBN 1572304995, 9781572304994.

Martin RWY, Ogston SA, Evans JR. Effects of vitamin and mineral supplementation on symptoms associated with chronic fatigue syndrome with Coxsackie B antibodies. *J Nutr Med.* 1994;4:11-23.

McDermott C, Richards SC, Thomas PW, et al. A placebo-controlled, double-blind, randomized controlled trial of a natural killer cell stimulant (BioBran MGN-3) in chronic fatigue syndrome. *QIM.* 2006 Jun 29 [Epub ahead of print].

McKenzie R, O'Fallon A, Dale J et al. (1998). "Low-dose hydrocortisone for treatment of chronic fatigue syndrome: a randomized controlled trial". *JAMA* **280 (12):** 1061-6. doi:10.1001/jama.280.12.1061 (http://dx.doi.org/10.1001%2Fjama.280.12.1061). PMID 9757853 (http://www.ncbi.nlm.nih.gov/pubmed/9757853).

Moss-Morris R, Hamilton W (April 2010). "Pragmatic rehabilitation for chronic fatigue syndrome" (http://eprints.soton.ac.uk/147139/2/bmj.c1799). *BMJ* **340:** c1799. doi:10.1136/bmj.c1799 (http://dx.doi.org/10.1136%2Fbmj.c1799). PMID 20418252 (http://www .ncbi .nlm.nih.gov/pubmed/20418252). http://eprints.soton.ac.uk/147139/2/bmj.c1799.

Moss-Morris R, Sharon C, Tobin R, Baldi JC (March 2005). "A randomized controlled graded exercise trial for chronic fatigue syndrome: outcomes and mechanisms of change". *J Health Psycho!* **10** (2): 245-59.

doi:10.1177/1359105305049774
(http://dx.doi.org/10.1177%2F1359105305049774) . PMID 15723894
(http://www.ncbi.nlm.nih.gov/pubmed/15723894).

Nasir JM, Durning SJ, Ferguson M, et al. Exercise-induced syncope associated
with QT prolongation and ephedra free Xenadrine. Mayo Clin Proc 2004;79:1059-
62.

Nijs J, Meeus M, De Meirleir K (August 2006). "Chronic musculoskeletal pain in
chronic fatigue syndrome: recent developments and therapeutic implications".
Man Ther **11 (3):** 187-91. doi:10.1016/j.math.2006.03.008
(http://dx.doi.org/10.1016%2Fj.math.2006.03.008) . PMID 16781183
(http://www.ncbi.nlm.nih.gov/pubmed/16781183)

Nijs J, Paul L, Wallman K (April 2008). "Chronic fatigue syndrome: an approach
combining self-management with graded exercise to avoid exacerbations". *J
Rehabil Med* **40** (4): 241-7. doi:10.2340/16501977-0185
(http://dx.doi.org/10.2340%2F16501977-0185) . PMID 18382818
(http://www.ncbi.nlm.nih.gov/pubmed/18382818).

Nunez M, Fernandez-Sola J, Nufiez E, Fernandez-Huerta JM, Godas-Sieso T,
Gomez-Gil E (January 2011). "Health-related quality of life in patients with
chronic fatigue syndrome: group cognitive behavioral therapy and graded
exercise versus usual treatment. A randomized controlled trial with 1 year of
follow-up". *Clin Rheumatol* **[Epub ahead of print]** (3): 381-9. doi:10.1007/s10067-
010-1677-y (http://dx.doi.org/10.1007%2Fs10067-010-1677-y) . PMID 21234629
(http://www .ncbi .nlm.nih.gov/pubmed/21234629) .

Nykamp DL, Fackih MN, Compton AL. Possible association of acute lateral-wall
myocardial infarction and bitter orange supplement. Ann Pharmacother
2004;38:812-6.

Op 't Eijnde B, Van Leemputte M, Brouns F, et al. No effects of oral ribose
supplementation on repeated maximal exercise and de novo ATP resynthesis. J
Appl Physiol 2001;9112275-81.

p. 13.
http://www.afme.org.uldres/img/resources/Survey%20Summary%20Report%
202008.pdf. Retrieved 8 March 2010.

Pae CU, Marks DM, Patkar AA, Masand PS, Luyten P, Serretti A (July 2009). "Pharmacological treatment of chronic fatigue syndrome: focusing on the role of antidepressants". *Expert Opin Pharmacother* **10** (10): 1561-70. doi:10.1517/14656560902988510 (http://dx.doi.org/10.1517%2F14656560902988510) . PMID 19514866 (http://www .ncbi .nlm.nih.gov/pubmed/19514866).

Plioplys AV, Plioplys S. Amantadine and L-carnitine treatment of chronic fatigue syndrome. *Neuropsychobiology.* 1997;35:16-23.

Price JR, Mitchell E, Tidy E, Hunot V (2008). Price, Jonathan R. ed. "Cognitive behavior therapy for chronic fatigue syndrome in adults". *Cochrane Database Syst Rev* (3): CD001027. doi:10.1002/14651858.CD001027.pub2 (http://dx.doi.org/10.1002%2F14651858.CD001027.pub2) . PMID 18646067 (http://www.ncbi.nlm.nih.gov/pubmed/18646067) .

Rea T, Buchwald D. Hydrocortisone and chronic fatigue syndrome [letter]. *Lancet.* 1999;353:1618-1619. Shepherd C. Hydrocortisone and chronic fatigue syndrome [letter]. *Lancet.* 1999;353:1619-1620.

Ridsdale L, Godfrey E, Chalder T et al. (January 2001). "Chronic fatigue in general practice: is counseling as good as cognitive behavior therapy? A UK randomized trial" (http://openurlingenta.com/content/nlm?genre=article&issn=0960-1643&volume=51&issue=462&spage=19&aulast=Ridsdale) . *Br J Gen Pract* **51** (462): 19 24. PMC 1313894 (http://www.pubmedcentral.gov/articlerenderfcgi?tool=pmcentrez&artid=1313894) .

Rimes KA, Chalder T. (2005). "Treatments for chronic fatigue syndrome." *Occupational Medicine* 55 (1): 32-39. doi:10.1093/occmedikqi015 (http://dx.doi.org/10.1093%2Foccmed%2Fkqi015) . PMID 15699088 (http://www.ncbi.nlm.nih.gov/pubmed/15699088) .

Rowe PC, Calkins H, DeBusk K, et al. Fludrocortisone acetate to treat neurally mediated hypotension in chronic fatigue syndrome: a randomized controlled trial. JAMA 2001;285:52-9.

Russmann S, Lauterberg BH, Helbling A. Kava hepatotoxicity [letter]. Ann Intern Med 2001;135:68-9. 7086 Liver Toxicity with kava. Pharmacist's Letter/Prescriber's Letter 2001;18(1):180115.

Sanders P, Korf J (2008). "Neuroaetiology of chronic fatigue syndrome: an overview". *World J. Biol. Psychiatry* **9 (3):** 165-71. doi:10.1080/15622970701310971 (http://dx.doi.org/10.1080%2F15622970701310971) . PMID 17853290 (http://www.ncbi.nlm.nih.gov/pubmed/17853290).

See DM, Broumand N, Sahl L, et al. In vitro effects of echinacea and ginseng on natural killer and antibody-dependent cell cytotoxicity in healthy subjects and chronic fatigue syndrome or acquired immunodeficiency patients. *Immunopharmacology.* 1997;35:229-235.

Smith S, Sullivan K. Examining the influence of biological and psychological factors on cognitive performance in chronic fatigue syndrome: a randomized, double-blind, placebo-controlled, crossover study. *Int J Behav Med.* 2003;10:162-173.

Stevens DL. Chronic fatigue. West J Med 2001;175:315-19.

Stewart JM. Autonomic nervous system dysfunction in adolescents with postural orthostatic tachycardia syndrome and chronic fatigue syndrome is characterized by attenuated vagal baroreflex and potentiated sympathetic vasomotion. Pediatr Res 2000;48:218-26.

Straus SE, Dale JK, Tobi M et al. (December 1988). "Acyclovir treatment of the chronic fatigue syndrome. Lack of efficacy in a placebo-controlled trial". *N. Engl. J. Med.* **319** (26): 1692-8. doi:10.1056/NEJM198812293192602 (http://dx.doi.org/10.1056%2FNEJM198812293192602) . PMID 2849717 (http://www .ncbi .nlm.nih.gov/pubmed/2849717).

Straus SE. History of chronic fatigue syndrome. Rev Infect Dis 1991;13:S2-S7. 10713 Reid S, Chalder T, Cleare A, et al. Chronic fatigue syndrome. BMJ 2000;320:292-6.

Teitelbaum JE, Johnson C, St Cyr J. The use of D-ribose in chronic fatigue syndrome and fibromyalgia: a pilot study. J Altern Complement Med 2006;12:857-62.

Twisk FN, Maes M (August 2009). "A review on cognitive behavioral therapy (CBT) and graded exercise therapy (GET) in myalgic encephalomyelitis (ME) / chronic fatigue syndrome (ME/CFS): CBT/GET is not only ineffective and not evidence-based, but also potentially harmful for many patients with ME/ME/CFS" (http://node.nel.edu/?node_id=8918) . *Neuro Endocrinol Lett* **30** (3): 284-299. PMID 19855350 (http://www.ncbi.nlm.nih.gov/pubmed/19855350).

Van Houdenhove B, Pae CU, Luyten P. Chronic fatigue syndrome: is there a role for non-antidepressant pharmacotherapy? Expert Opin Pharmacother 2010;11:215-23.

Vermeulen RC, Scholte HR. Exploratory open label, randomized study of acetyl- and propionylcarnitine in chronic fatigue syndrome. Psychosom Med 2004;66:276-82.

Wallman KE, Morton AR, Goodman C, Grove R, Guilfoyle AM (May 2004). "Randomized controlled trial of graded exercise in chronic fatigue syndrome" (http://www .mja.com.au/public/issues/18009_030504/wal10613_fm.html) . *Med. J. Aust.* **180** (9): 444-8. PMID 15115421 (http://www.ncbi.nlm.nih.gov/pubmed/15115421).

Warren G, McKendrick M, Peet M (1999). "The role of essential fatty acids in chronic fatigue syndrome. A case-controlled study of red-cell membrane essential fatty acids (EFA) and a placebo-controlled treatment study with high dose of EFA". *Acta Neurol. Scand.* **99** (2): 112-6. doi:10.1111/j.1600-0404.1999.tb00667.x (http://dx.doi.org/10.1111%2Fj.1600-0404.1999.tb00667.x). PMID 10071170 (http://www.ncbi.nlm.nih.gov/pubmed/10071170).

Wiborg JF, Knoop **H,** Stulemeijer M, Prins JB, Bleijenberg G (January 2010). "How does cognitive behaviour therapy reduce fatigue in patients with chronic fatigue syndrome? The role of physical activity". *Psychol Med* **40** (8): 1-7. doi:10.1017/S0033291709992212 (http://dx.doi.org/10.1017%2FS0033291709992212) . PMID 20047707

Williams G, Waterhouse J, Mugarza J, et al. Therapy of circadian rhythm disorders in chronic fatigue syndrome: no symptomatic improvement with melatonin or phototherapy. *EurJ Clin Invest* 2002;32:831 837.

Wilson A, Hickie I, Lloyd A, et al. Longitudinal study of outcome of chronic fatigue syndrome. BMJ 1994;308:756-9. 10723 Natelson BH. Chronic fatigue syndrome. JAMA 2001;285:2557-9.

Yiu YM, Ng SM, Tsui YL, et al. A clinical trial of acupuncture for treating chronic fatigue syndrome in Hong Kong.] *Zhong Xi Yi Jie He Xue Bao.* 2007;5:630-633.